A Big Glass of Water

Surviving Throat Cancer and Treatment
My Journey

JEFF DANZIK, LCSW
LICENSED CLINICAL SOCIAL WORKER
AND THROAT CANCER SURVIVOR

ISBN: 9781701637665

Book Layout and Design by Sarco Press

Life is, has always been, and will always be, extremely fragile. The only thing that changes is our perception of this fact.

- Jeff Danzik

To my wife, Angela.
I don't know if I would have made it through
this journey without your love and support.
I am eternally grateful.

ACKNOWLEDGEMENTS

There are people who touch our lives, however briefly or infrequently, who leave imprints on our souls. I am lucky that I have been touched by many of these angels.

To my friend Fredrick von Tress who lost his battle with cancer just as I was beginning mine. We joked about sitting side by side and chatting all day as we began chemotherapy treatments together. He never made it to his. I miss his sense of humor, his openness, and his guidance.

To Valerie Niestrath who was one of the gentlest beings I have ever known. She was a teacher, a healer, and a friend. Her light radiated from her right up until she left us, succumbing to cancer.

To my mother, Barbara Danzik, who died five months before I knew I had cancer. It had been a long struggle for her, and I am glad she finally found peace.

To my father, Mitch Danzik, who died three days before I received my cancer diagnosis. He never knew I had cancer, and I am thankful he was spared the worry. We had always been father and son, but during the last year of his life, we had finally become friends. I am so thankful for that. I miss him every day.

To Jennifer Lewellyn, Rachel Cicerrella, and Gail Kessler who may or may not know this, but along with my wife, were my morale and mental health team. They were the ones who kept me going when I wanted to give up.

Jennifer was there for me from the beginning until the end and beyond, and her support and kindness were and are appreciated beyond words. She has made a friend for life.

Rachel's sense of humor, positive outlook, and genuineness helped me become a little less lost inside of my own egoic despair. I looked forward to and enjoyed our time together.

Gail's strength, stability, and ability to listen without flinching was so helpful for me. I looked forward to our time and believed that simply being in her presence was healing for me.

To Dr. Aleksandra Sander, M.D. who was the ONLY medical professional to ever tell me that I would be okay. I continue to be amazed by her. She handles so much and deals with so many people who are dying and in pain, and yet she smiles, connects, is present, and genuinely cares about others. She was one of those who was pivotal in saving my life. Thank you for that.

To Dr. Joseph Clark, M.D. who found my cancer, and was relentless at getting to the truth about where it had spread in spite of others having differing opinions. He made sure my diagnosis was clear so that I would receive the correct treatment. He was gentle, kind, and honest. He was also pivotal in saving my life. Thank you.

To Dr. Celisha Gerber, N.D. who identified issues, imparted information to me, and guided me on a course that no Western doctor would have. I am sure that without her help, my recovery would have taken much longer and may not have been as successful. She is a kind and gentle soul, and I am lucky to have found her.

Thank you to Lillian and the group at Providence Infusion for their diligence and follow up. Thank you to the physicians, staff, technicians, and nurses at Hematology Oncology

Associates and the Dubs Cancer Center, who do impossible jobs day in and day out. And thank you to my friends and family who supported me. The cards, emails, and messages meant so much to me.

I also want to thank those who helped me with proofing and editing this book: Joe Spurgeon, Richard Boucher, Kate Mole, Mike Rulon, Jeff Fayerharm, Chuck Katz, Kimberly McMartin, and Michele Mathews. They all helped me by reviewing my writing, catching mistakes, and suggesting changes. Their assistance was very much appreciated.

Thank you to Glenn Bontrager at Sarco Press for working with me on my book layout and design, tolerating my edits and changes, and helping me to make this book available in print and ebook formats.

Lastly, I want to acknowledge all of those who have experienced or continue to experience cancer and express my gratitude to those who care for them.

x

CONTENTS

Introduction 1

PART 1

Chapter 1: Suggestions to Consider When Beginning
the Cancer Process 13

Chapter 2: Diagnosis (PART 1) 27

Chapter 3: My Crisis of Faith 31

Chapter 4: Diagnosis (PART 2)-Further Diagnostic Testing ..35

Chapter 5: Preparation for Treatment 43

Chapter 6: Treatment 59

Chapter 7: My Friend the Feeding Tube 79

Chapter 8: Recovery 101

Chapter 9: Side Effects and Annoyances After Treatment 111

Chapter 10: Recommendations During Recovery 123

Chapter 11: The Financial Impact 131

PART II

Chapter 12: The Psychological Impact of Dealing
with Cancer 139

Chapter 13: Grief 147

Chapter 14: Trauma 153

Chapter 15: Suggestions for Caring for your Emotional Health .167

Chapter 16: Recommendations for System Change 175

Chapter 17: Compassion 179

Chapter 18: Gratitude and Giving Back 191

Epilogue 195

Appendix 1 199

Appendix 2 205

INTRODUCTION

M Y NAME IS Jeff Danzik, and I am a throat cancer survivor. I assume you are reading this because you or someone close to you has been diagnosed with throat cancer or a similar type. I am sorry. Receiving a cancer diagnosis and participating in treatment are traumatic, life-changing events. There is no way to escape this reality. The good news is that cancers of the throat and/or mouth are usually treatable with a high percentage of successful outcomes.

On August 30, 2017, I received my official cancer diagnosis—P-16, HPV positive, squamous cell carcinoma of my epiglottis with right lymph node involvement. I had throat cancer. Several small tumors had grown where my tongue met my throat, and the cancer had spread to a few lymph nodes on the right side of my neck. I was fifty-four years old and in excellent health. I had only smoked briefly in my twenties and had never been exposed (as far as I was aware) to any carcinogenic chemicals. I had been running again, attending an exercise class a few nights a week, eating a healthy diet, and losing a few pounds. Life was good. How could I have throat cancer?

I decided to write about my experience for two reasons. First, I hope to help you or someone you know deal with the diagnosis, treatment, and recovery from what the medical profession classifies as "head and neck cancer". Though my experience was with throat cancer, I hope that some of the information I share is helpful for anyone dealing with any type of cancer.

Cancer is scary. The medical community focuses on the diagnoses, physical effects, and treatment of this disease. They tend to overlook the emotional needs of cancer patients. If there is even one thing in this book that makes the cancer process a little easier for you or someone close to you, I have achieved my goal. I had to learn many things for myself along the way, and I wish I had someone to tell me some of these things before I learned the hard way. I hope the story of my cancer journey can provide useful information, ideas, and resources as you or someone you know goes through their journey.

Second, I have written this book for my own psychological healing. Telling my story has helped me process my own emotions around my cancer experience. As I will mention several times, the majority of cancer treatment does not address the emotional component of dealing with this disease.

This opinion is based on my experience as a patient and as a professional. I am a licensed clinical social worker and have a private practice where I work as a psychotherapist. Though I have not had a great deal of experience working with cancer patients in my career, I have worked for many years with individuals with disabilities and with those who experienced trauma in their lives.

I am not a physician, and what I write is not intended to be medical advice. It is also not intended to be all-inclusive in any way. This is simply my experience, my opinion, and what worked and didn't work for me. I would like to think that due to my experience and my profession that I do have some knowledge about the psychological aspects of disease and trauma. I also provide information I discovered while doing my own research. I hope there is something I have learned that can help you.

I finished my treatment on November 30, 2017. So far, I remain cancer free. I had contemplated writing my story for a long time but was not sure I was prepared to deal with the feelings that putting my experience on paper would evoke, and honestly, as I write this, I still wonder if I am ready.

I have divided my cancer experience into four significant phases: diagnosis, preparation, treatment, and recovery. These phases are only for reference, and there may be some overlap. Categorizing the phases of my experience helped me to track what was happening and helped me to better understand the process. It also helped me determine some milestones to antic-ipate along the way. Classifying the phases in this way helped me to better communicate with medical professionals and other patients. Sometimes confusion would arise from using the same words but having different definitions of what they might mean.

The year I was diagnosed with throat cancer was a rough year. After a long decline from dementia and kidney failure, my mother died five months before I was diagnosed. Unexpectedly, my father died three days before my official cancer diagnosis. Neither one of my parents ever knew I had cancer.

Soon after I was diagnosed, a good friend of mine was told that he had terminal bone cancer, and he died a few weeks after I started treatment. These events impacted me greatly as well.

I have not even attempted to distinguish the psychological impact of my cancer and treatment from the psychological impact of the other losses that occurred during that year. However, I do acknowledge that given the number of signif-icant losses I experienced within a short span of time, it is quite possible that my recovery (at least psychologically) has been more difficult than if I was only dealing with recovering from cancer and treatment. During the entire diagnosis, preparation, and treatment process, there were so many things to focus on that there was little room for me to grieve my other losses. It wasn't until I was some months into recovery that I really began to grieve. I am still working through all of it.

In the end, I am not sure if being able to separate what impacted me more makes a difference or not. My story is my story, and we all have our different, unique experiences. There is never "a good time" to find out you have cancer. There is never a "good time" to go through treatment. Cancer does not discriminate. It doesn't care how old you are, what race you are, if you are straight or gay, if you are religious or not, how much money you make, or what else is going on in your life at the time. It simply shows up and demands attention.

Yet I had never experienced my cancer as the problem. I had a scratchy throat. That was all. It felt minor. Before treatment I never had difficulty eating, swallowing, or tasting food. I never felt sick or excessively tired. The issues I experienced and the problems I had and continue to have both physically and psychologically are a result of treatment. They are not the result of the cancer.

This feels odd to me since there is no doubt in my mind that left untreated, the cancer would have killed me, probably within six months, and it would have been an unpleasant way to die. This "reality" contradicted my experience before and after diagnosis, where I felt fine until treatment began. It is still something that is hard for me to digest at times. I felt fine with cancer, but it would have soon killed me. I felt terrible during treatment, but it saved my life.

I have noticed that many of my thoughts and feelings about my cancer process are often contradictory. Western medicine saved my life. At the same time, there were issues and experiences I had with Western medicine that I am angry and resentful about. Overall, I received amazing care, but it was lacking in some significant areas.

I still have not resolved many of these contradictory emotions and realize I may never be able to do so. You will undoubtedly see this reflected in my writing. The cancer process is full of highs and lows. It only makes sense that my thoughts and emotions would follow that path as well.

Dealing with cancer changes a person both physically and psychologically. I don't believe there is any way that it cannot. There is nothing as profound as facing our own mortality. Cancer is a traumatic life event, and the impact does not go away when treatment ends. I don't believe the impact ever goes away. We learn to live with a new normal. Our identity changes. What was important will likely change. Goals and priorities and our perceived purpose in life will likely change. Even our belief in whatever higher power we ascribe to (or don't ascribe to) will be called into question.

How the trauma of cancer and treatment impacts you and those around you will depend on several things: your basic personality type, the ways in which you cope with things, and the support system you have and create. The type and location of your cancer, the prognosis, the duration and type of treatment, the severity of side effects, the outcome of your treatment, the lifestyle changes that may be necessary, and your physical health, will all impact how you deal with the cancer process both physically and psychologically. There also seems to be a random component to this equation. Sometimes things just happen, and we don't know why. They cannot be predicted, like being diagnosed with throat cancer in the first place.

The process from diagnosis to recovery was not easy. And yet there are many positive things I gleaned from the experience. I would like to believe that the whole experience of cancer and treatment has made me a better person. It has helped me prioritize what is and isn't important in this life. I created unexpected friendships with some of the people I met who were part of my process, and I know they will be friends for life. I met people (other patients and professionals) who I may never see again, but I will always remember and appreciate them. I deepened relationships with friends and acquaintances who I would have never expected to step forward to help and support me. My relationship with my wife strengthened, and we bonded on a level that I believe only could have happened when being forced to deal with a life-threatening illness. I also finally lost the weight I wanted to lose. I tell people that the cancer diet is extremely effective, but I wouldn't recommend it!

In a strange and twisted way, part of me is thankful for the experience. And I NEVER want to repeat it. I am different now—hopefully in a better way. I would like to believe that I am more compassionate and more present. I am still in the process of reorganizing my values and priorities in life. I have a strong desire to give something back to this world. I highly doubt I would be experiencing these things as intensely or as mindfully without going through my experience with cancer.

Many of the side effects of treatment I was told would occur, I never experienced. Other side effects I did experience. I also experienced physical and psychological issues no one ever told me about or others who have gone through this treatment never had to deal with. This is part of what is so hard about cancer, treatment, and recovery. Each experience can be quite different.

I only intimately know my own experience. I was diagnosed with throat cancer, and I could see the tumors in my throat. I was told the cancer was aggressive and fast growing and had spread to at least one, maybe two, lymph nodes on the right side of my neck. It had not spread anywhere else. My treatment was six weeks of weekly chemotherapy sessions (one full day per week for six weeks) and thirty-three daily (Monday – Friday) radiation treatments to my throat and neck. I needed to use a feeding tube soon after treatment began and used it exclusively to eat for five months, meaning that for five months I could not eat by mouth. Soon after I began treatment, I also received IV hydration for two hours per day, six days a week, for two months.

During my cancer process, I went to urgent care once with problems with my skin around the feeding tube. I spent another evening in the emergency room due to feeding tube issues and dehydration, and I had a three-day hospital stay after treatment ended due to developing a fever likely caused by chemotherapy.

My treatment was successful. I no longer have any detectable cancer in my body, and the tumors in my throat are gone. I have a few lingering side effects that may or may not go away, but I can eat and drink again and basically do everything that I could do before my diagnosis and treatment. I will only have to deal with some minor physical issues for the rest of my life (e.g. some swelling in my neck, taste bud changes, thyroid damage from radiation, and some hearing loss from the chemotherapy drug). I also have experienced and continue to experience the emotional impact of what I went through. I will likely always deal with some issues related to my cancer and treatment, but I am confident that the intensity will lessen with time and help.

Please know that you are not alone. There are thousands of people who have had this disease and thousands who have survived it. There is support available. You might have to actively seek it out for yourself, but it is there.

I hope my experience can help you make decisions or at least help you ask questions. Doctors are not always right, and Western medicine does not necessarily have all of the answers. There is no clear map for navigating this journey, and it is often not a straightforward linear process. In the end, I had to make the final decisions regarding my care and recovery and had a great many things to consider. In the end, I had to trust my own intuition and judgment as to what the right path was for me. There is no "right" way to do all of this, and there are many options. Making what feels like the right choice for you may not be an easy thing.

Just as no two people are alike, no two cancers or cancer experiences are alike. Changes and problems will occur, but the impact, intensity, and discomfort will vary for each individual. The physical and psychological effects, short-term and long-term, will also vary. Again, there is no formula here. However, I do believe you can influence the outcome. Your physical and psychological condition before, during, and after treatment can make a huge contribution toward a successful recovery.

Some people will want to know every aspect of the process they are about to go through, including every possible outcome, side effect, and treatment option. Others become overwhelmed easily and don't want too much information at once. What I have written is the sum of my experience and information that I have gathered since the beginning of my journey. It can be overwhelming to digest all at once. It is still overwhelming for me at times. You can read everything I have written now, or you can read it in parts and pieces over time. I have tried to break things down so that you will know where there is a particular topic you may want to read about.

The first section of this book focuses on the physical aspects of cancer and treatment. Included in this are all of my experiences of being diagnosed, preparing for treatment, participating in treatment, and recovering from treatment. The second section of this book deals with the psychological aspects of my experience, something that is not talked about much by medical professionals but is addressed in support groups and individual and group therapy.

There are always those who have it easier and those who have it harder. Classifying my own or someone else's experience as being better or worse than yours might not be helpful. Though I have wanted to compare my experience to others, I have found no value in doing this. It only led to me feeling guilty that I made it through relatively unscathed compared to others. Your experience will be your experience. It may or may not be similar to my experience or the experience of the person next to you. However, I would like to think the suggestions I make could be helpful in creating the best possible experience with the least amount of suffering.

Another thing to consider when making decisions throughout your process is that cancer is a hugely profitable business. I can't help but question how this impacts every aspect of the process. As of 2018, the cancer industry makes over $100 billion dollars per year. My medical costs were estimated to have been between $225,000 and $250,000. This included all testing, procedures, pharmaceuticals, physician and clinic visits, hospitalizations, and feeding tube formula and supplies. I have yet to factor in the cost of recovery, which includes follow up visits, medications, psychological help, and meeting with other professionals who are now involved in my life as part of my ongoing effort to stay healthy.

There are two main cancer treatment centers where I live. The first is a radiation oncology clinic where a cancer patient receives radiation treatments. The second is a medical oncology clinic where patients receive their chemotherapy treatments.

The radiation oncology clinic in my community is owned and operated by a nonprofit organization. They have a staff of radiological oncologists, radiological technicians, a social worker, and a nurse navigator—whose job is to help patients navigate the system and assist with any issue that may occur related to their cancer. The clinic is always busy and always seems understaffed.

The medical oncology clinic here is owned and operated by one of the largest medical corporations in the country, McKesson Corporation. They are a for-profit company who sells the drugs and most of the equipment used in the clinic. They also supply pharmaceuticals to over half of the hospitals in the United States. The clinic here employs several medical oncologists. They have their own laboratory and staff and have several chemotherapy nurses, technicians, and other staff. The medical oncology clinic easily has two to three times the number of staff that the radiology clinic has. Yet, at present, they have no social workers and no nurse navigators on staff. They offer no psychological services of any kind, not even information and/ or referral. During a chemotherapy education workshop that I was required to attend, the psychological impact of cancer treatment was never mentioned, while every possible physical side effect of the treatment was discussed at length.

You can draw your own conclusions from this information. It is hard for me to believe that money and profits do not significantly impact care, including what care is recommended, and the quality of care. What exactly that impact is or how that impact affects you directly, I leave it for you to decide.

PART 1

CHAPTER 1
SUGGESTIONS TO CONSIDER WHEN BEGINNING THE CANCER PROCESS

THERE ARE MANY things I wish I would have known as I started my cancer process. Here is a list of some suggestions based on my experience.

1. Talk to friends, doctors, patients, social workers, and naturopaths. Get multiple opinions, ask a lot of questions, and trust your intuition.

You can find a great deal of information about cancer and treatment. Some of it may be contradictory. I wish I would have talked to more people in the beginning or sought out more advice from other medical professionals (e.g. a naturopath) and others who have been through this treatment. I would not have changed my choice about completing chemotherapy and radiation treatments, but there were things along the way (which I will discuss later) that I would have done differently had I known then what I know now. Some of what I learned came from my own experience, and some of it I obtained by talking to others who had completed treatment (I should have talked to other survivors sooner).

2. Find a support group as soon as possible. They are a great resource.

There is a national organization that provides support for individuals who have head and neck cancer (The medical profession considers throat cancer as part of the classification of "head and neck cancer".). The organization is called SPOHNC (Support for People with Oral, Head, and Neck Cancer) and their website is www.spohnc.org. They have local chapters in most areas. They have a wealth of information on their website, including information on local chapters that offer support groups.

I wish I would have connected with this group before beginning treatment or at least used this resource to connect with an individual who had been through treatment. The national chapter even has a mentoring program which will match you up with someone who has been through a similar experience. Talking to someone who has survived treatment, is able to answer questions and support you, can be invaluable. The only caution is making sure you are comfortable with the person or group, which leads me to my next suggestion.

3. Be CLEAR about what you want and don't want.

Being clear applies to support, treatment, and even information. I made the choice to use Facebook as a support tool for my treatment. I posted about my cancer and treatment. I was very clear that I did not want my Facebook friends suggesting alternative treatments or telling me stories about their friend or relative who had cancer. I only wanted people to ask how I was doing and, if they could, offer to help (with things like shopping, transportation, etc., if I needed it). I certainly didn't want to hear any stories about people dying of cancer, becoming disfigured, or the like. I only wanted the information I wanted at the time that was relevant to what was happening that moment, not information about what might be happening week three of treatment or week six or the second month after. Some people may want to hear suggestions or stories. I knew it would not work for me.

4. Train for treatment.

I was diagnosed on August 30, 2017. My first radiation treatment was October 16th and my first chemotherapy treatment was about a week after that. I didn't experience any side effects until the beginning of November. So, it was about two months between my diagnosis and when I started experiencing the first side effects of treatment.

Before treatment begins and as long as you are able, I would suggest taking the best care of yourself possible. Doing what you can to get your body and mind in shape for the next phases can help lessen its impact and help recovery.

My recommendations would include exercising, eating well, lowering your stress level, and whatever else you can do to get your body and mind prepared. I looked at this as training and as if my life depended on it. My wife often equated making it through treatment to running a marathon, which I had done once in 2005. I trained for it for about eight months.

Being in good physical and psychological shape is a great way to give yourself the best chance of minimizing side effects (both physical and psychological) and the best chance for recovery. I whole-heartedly believe that because I was in good shape physically and mentally prior to the start of treatment that it greatly contributed to my recovery.

I would suggest not concentrating on weight loss before treatment even if it is needed. I know very few people who have made it through treatment without losing weight, and weight loss during treatment is something doctors do not like. I was told more than once that those who have the best success in recovering from treatment are those who can keep weight on during treatment. If weight loss is needed, it should be done after treatment and healing is complete. That being said, I lost thirty-five pounds during treatment over about three months. I received a stern lecture and even had my team do an "intervention" to get me to take in more calories. In spite of that, I have kept off most of the weight I had lost, which, for me, is a good thing because I needed to lose some weight, and it DID NOT impede my recovery at all. So, this is something, like so many things during cancer treatment and recovery, that can vary from person to person, and you have to make your own choices regarding this.

5. Keep a journal.

Keeping a journal was invaluable for me. The amount of information you will receive can be overwhelming. Handling it in a state of shock, anger, or grief is even harder. I knew NOTHING about throat cancer, nothing about treatment, and not much about cancer of any type. Everything was new, and my life depended on the information I was receiving and the questions I might ask. Keeping everything in one place was necessary and convenient. I wrote down information, questions, concerns, appointments, to-do lists, my feelings, and anything and everything related to cancer, treatment, and recovery. There was no way I could rely on my memory.

There are no rules about how a journal is kept. It can be an outlet for difficult emotions, a place to keep recipes and food cravings (when it became hard to eat, I started dreaming of food), or where you can list all of the things you appreciate and have to look forward to in the future.

6. Stay positive or as positive as you can.

Staying positive can be difficult. Being overwhelmed is normal. Being angry, sad, or resentful are all normal. Feeling optimistic one minute and fearing death the next is normal. Being numb and/or being hypersensitive is normal. All is normal. There is no wrong way to think, feel, act, or be. It all will likely feel crazy at times, and yes, this is normal too.

I strongly believe that your mindset during this journey is extremely important. This does not mean that you won't be sad or angry at times but accepting what is happening is extremely important. Your mindset is not something that will likely be discussed much by the professionals involved in your cancer process.

It has been said that suffering can be defined as a refusal to accept reality for what it is. I sincerely believe this. When I was diagnosed with cancer, my reality changed. My life changed.

Before starting treatment, I closed my practice and stopped working. During treatment I saw some type of doctor or medical professional almost daily. I couldn't eat and had to rely on a feeding tube. My appearance changed, and sometimes I didn't even recognize myself. My life became focused around treatment and recovery.

The more I refused to accept this, the more I added to my suffering. Energy spent fighting against reality is wasted energy. And we all do it. Again, I didn't have to like it or be happy about it, but refusing to accept it just caused more pain.

7. Find a mental health therapist.

There is no question that cancer is a physical assault on the body. It is also an assault on the mind. Unfortunately, this is still something that Western medicine, overall, does not address. I was facing my own mortality. I was looking at treatment with all its difficulties and possible long-term effects. I was in disbelief, angry, scared, sad, and frustrated. Sometimes I would feel all these emotions within the span of a few minutes. Experiencing a cancer diagnosis and everything that goes with it is a traumatic event. Our psychological reaction needs to be assessed and treated as well as our body.

The medical professionals I saw did not address the psychological aspects of cancer. It was not until later that I discovered that the radiation oncologist's office had a social worker and a nurse navigator on staff. The nurse navigator was the person who answered any question or helped with any need I had. She would either direct me to the right person, advocate for me, help coordinate a service, or figure out the answer for me. These two people helped save my life as much as the medical doctors did.

I have a friend who developed cancer that had spread to her colon, liver, and stomach. She had to have part of her colon removed, was on radiation for a few months, and now has been on chemotherapy for over two years. She will have to use a colostomy bag for the rest of her life. Her exact prognosis is not known though it doesn't look great. She is in and out of the hospital.

She talks about wanting to find ways to feel more positive. She asks others how to stop feeling depressed and talks a great deal about how to distract herself from what is happening to her. Yet she refuses to discuss seeing a therapist or going to a support group. When I bring this up to her, she does not respond and changes the subject.

I don't understand this at all. Her cancer impacted her body and caused problems, so she sought out treatment. Her same cancer and treatment are impacting her psyche and causing problems, so why not seek out treatment for that?

I am going to step up on my soapbox for a moment. If

you have never in your life had a problem that you couldn't deal with yourself, I still recommend a therapist. If you believe that therapy is for the weak, which, of course, I believe is not true, I would encourage you to talk about this with a therapist. If you want to heal from this disease and embrace life again, I recommend a therapist. There might be physical scars at the end of treatment. There will likely be emotional ones. For these to heal, you will probably need help with psychological healing just as you did for your physical healing. It doesn't have to be forever and could help speed up recovery.

This is as applicable for caregivers of cancer patients as it is for the patient, especially if the caregiver is a spouse or family member. The trauma of cancer and treatment is not limited only to the patient.

If people were generally able to heal their own psychological problems, my profession would no longer be needed. In fact, in my experience, the more resistant someone is to receiving psychological help when there is an emotional problem and the more that person insists "I can handle it myself," the slower and more difficult recovery becomes. Okay, I'm stepping off my soapbox now.

For me personally, I already knew a great deal about trauma and grief. In my practice, I help people deal with these issues on a daily basis. I could argue that since I knew this stuff, I didn't need outside help. Yet I knew enough to know that I did indeed need outside help. I still do. Trauma takes time to process. Psychological healing is usually much slower than physical healing and sometimes harder. I would estimate that I am at least ninety percent physically healed from cancer and treatment. I would estimate that I am about seventy percent healed from the psychological effects and have suffered from what is called an unspecified trauma disorder.

Cancer will change you. It will change the people close to

you. Complete healing must include the body and the mind. Most people would not try to treat their cancer themselves. Why would someone try to treat their own depression, anxiety, and/or trauma responses without professional help? Again, you have to make these decisions for yourself, but I know for me and my experience, psychological help through this process has been as valuable as physical assistance.

8. Find a point person.

I know people have different levels of support. I was very lucky to have a wonderful wife who cared for me. I don't know how I would have made it through all of this without her. I have also known people who must deal with all of this on their own without any support.

If it is available to you, find one person who is your "point" person. In my case it was my wife. She kept track of my appointments, attended appointments with me when she was able, took notes for me, and coordinated things when I could not. Everyone experiences treatment differently, but confusion generally becomes part of the process. I had never heard the term "chemo brain" before treatment, but now I understand it intimately. It is a kind of confusion and slightly altered state that is caused by chemotherapy treatment that has to be experienced to be fully understood. It is highly likely that a cancer patient will experience greater confusion during treatment. Having someone as a "point" person can be a life saver—literally.

If it can't be one person, see if you can spread out the responsibilities. My wife and I sat down and made a list of people who we could ask to help with certain things. This could include transportation, research, making appointments, or sitting with me. We had over thirty people on our list.

To my surprise and appreciation, many people offered to help without being asked. You will discover that some people in your life are better friends than you ever thought they were. Some people will send cards, call you, and do things for you. And some people will disappear from your life. I wouldn't take this personally if it happens. Most people in our culture are not comfortable with anything that reminds them of their own mortality. We typically don't talk about death. I chose to look at those who disappeared from my life as scared to face the reality that all life ends.

9. Be discerning about what you read online.

I remember someone once telling me that when you have a good experience with something, you might tell others about it. However, if you have a bad experience with something, you will definitely share it with others. If you search the internet, it is easy to find every worst-case scenario of anything.

Soon after my diagnosis, I started reading cancer stories online. This was a HUGE mistake. I DO NOT recommend this. I remember reading a horrific account of what happened to a woman during treatment. It only served to terrify me, and I experienced nothing even close to what she did.

You will find every possible scenario online, most of which appear to be bad experiences. I did not find it helpful at all to read these. At one point, I even asked my wife if she would be willing to look up some stories online for me and share with me only positive outcomes. This was helpful.

As I explained before, I had also asked anyone who knew about my cancer not to tell me any negative stories about friends, relatives, or themselves as it related to cancer treatment. I only wanted suggestions regarding treatment or recovery from those who had been through it themselves, not from someone who read some article or heard about some study or treatment. I wanted positive in my life. Looking up cancer stories online was not positive.

This changed a little bit as treatment progressed. When a specific issue or question came up, I would sometimes look up information. I tried to be very specific in my searches or I would ask my wife to look something up for me.

How this impacts each person will vary. I know myself and my tendency to worry, so a self-imposed moratorium on internet use for cancer research was a wise choice. In fact, I didn't return to the internet for any information regarding cancer until several months after treatment ended, and even then, only for some of the specific information/and resources I needed to write this book.

10. Advocate for yourself.

This sounds like a simple, obvious thing. I have been employed as a client advocate before in my career, and yet in hindsight there were times during my cancer experience where I was not a very good advocate for myself. By giving up or getting angry and resisting some things or not resisting other things, I ended up making it harder for myself. I knew when things didn't feel right or make sense to me. Yet I often wouldn't trust my own intuition.

As I said, there is no clear, linear, agreed upon formula for all of this. You will find professional and lay people who are adamant about their point of view about what is right for you. Sometimes they will agree, and sometimes they won't. Sometimes the information or recommendations you receive will agree with your own beliefs, opinions, and values, or intuition, and sometimes they won't.

I wish I would have been more assertive about issues related to my feeding tube and formula. I wish I would have set clearer boundaries with the care I received when I was in the hospital or had refused to go in the first place. I wish I would have started seeing a naturopath at the beginning of my treatment and worked with him/her concurrently. I will talk more about these issues later.

I had gut feelings about all these things, but I didn't listen to myself and paid a price. It was my life and my responsibility to ultimately make decisions that I believed were best for me. This was not easy and often meant deciding things based on conflicting information. It also meant sometimes having conflict with professionals who, in my opinion, would have been much happier had I passively followed whatever path or treatment I was directed to take without question.

Ultimately, I did choose to do most of what was recommended to me, and I made some choices that were in addition to what I viewed as the "status quo" of treatment. Whatever I chose, I did my best to make an informed choice after talking to others, doing my own research, and soul searching. I had to decide who I trusted and who I didn't, and what I trusted and what I did not.

I can't tell you what is right for you. Some people will elect not to participate in all or parts of treatment. Some people will seek alternative treatments. And some people will go along with whatever the standard medical treatment of the day happens to be. What I am suggesting is that you become as involved as you can in your own decisions and advocate for what you believe is right for you as if your life depended on it. There is ultimately no single correct answer.

11. Don't believe everything you are told or everything you think.

There was a time in the past where a doctor's word was

law. People assumed doctors knew everything, and their advice should be followed without question. This does not seem to be the case anymore. In our current technological age, we have access to an overwhelming amount of sometimes contradictory information. Medicine is not nor has it ever been an exact science. Things are changing all the time. Whatever is the latest greatest treatment today, guaranteed to save your life, can easily become outdated or be viewed as barbaric in the future. Information, procedures, processes, and medications are constantly changing and what works for one individual may or may not work for another.

There was more than one instance when I was told something about my experience or believed something about my experience that was just plain wrong. Receiving radiation and chemotherapy and being on multiple medications opens the door to many potential side effects. It is often difficult to discern what caused what and why or even know what side effects I might experience.

Many of the side effects that I was experiencing (mainly feeling bad and being tired and nauseous all of the time) were attributed to the chemotherapy drug I was receiving. Some of this was true, but when I completed treatment, the assumption remained that the issues I continued to experience were a result of chemotherapy and radiation. This was not correct. I discovered that two major factors contributing to why I didn't feel well during and after treatment were my reaction to the feeding formula and being dehydrated.

There were indeed other contributors as well. I had become anemic. My white cell count was extremely low, and the combination of fentanyl and hydrocodone left me tired and less than lucid much of the time.

The reason this was important to sort out was so I could figure out how I might remedy the issue or issues that were causing me discomfort. After I began hydration, I felt a little better. When I changed my feeding formula, I felt much better and began recovering faster. If I had taken what I was told at face value, that all of my symptoms were a result of my treatment and rest was the only solution, my recovery would have been much slower.

CHAPTER 2
DIAGNOSIS (PART 1)

MISTAKENLY BELIEVED THAT receiving a cancer diagnosis was a clear and discernible single event. In the case of cancer, diagnosis is typically a process that involves several tests and procedures which eventually led to hearing those dreaded words, "You have cancer."

I saw two distinct parts to the diagnosis phase. The first was the definitive conclusion that I had cancer (the results of my biopsies and x-rays validated this). The second part was the definitive indication of where the cancer was, if it had spread, and where it had spread to. For me, the first phase of the diagnosis process began with a routine visit to my primary care physician for a physical. This led to X-rays of my thyroid and esophagus. When these showed nothing, I was referred to an ear, nose, and throat specialist (ENT).

Some cancers are found quite by accident or somehow discovered by a routine examination or test. However, sometimes there is an indication that something is not right. In my case, sometime before July 2017, I noticed I had a scratchy throat that wouldn't go away. This was my only symptom. When I first noticed this, I thought I was getting a cold. When it didn't go away and I didn't get sick, I knew there had to be some issue, but I figured it was minor and could wait. I had no cough, no pain, and no difficulty swallowing. I thought maybe I had a piece of food that had gotten caught under the tissue in my throat.

I have no idea if seeing a physician sooner would have changed anything. I do know that my cancer was aggressive. I have talked to survivors who knew something was wrong for a year or two before having it checked. The result of their procrastination was dealing with a more serious cancer process than they might have had if they had been checked sooner. It may be better to be safe and see a doctor if there is any suspicion of something not being right.

When I went in for my annual physical, I told my doctor about my scratchy throat, and he thought he felt something around my thyroid and ordered a thyroid X-ray. Nothing abnormal showed in the X-ray, but I still had a scratchy throat. The next thing he ordered was an X-ray of my esophagus. It was clear as well. Next was an appointment with an ENT.

The ENT used what is called a laryngoscope to look into my throat. It was a long cable with a small lens/mirror at the end of it that can project an image onto a screen. The ENT can insert this into your throat or nose, which threads into your throat, so it can be viewed on a screen. My ENT sprayed something in my nose to numb it a bit and inserted the cable up my nose. The procedure was a little uncomfortable, but not painful, and only lasted a few minutes. The view of my throat, which I could see projected onto a screen, showed several small tumors which he suspected were cancerous. To confirm his suspicion, I needed to have a biopsy done.

THROAT BIOPSY

The throat biopsy was a surgical procedure where I needed to be put to sleep. While asleep, the ENT cut a small sample of the tumors in my throat to be sent to the lab and examined to determine if they were cancerous. I did not feel any pain at all when I woke up. Evidently some people do, and others do not.

After I woke up from the throat biopsy, the doctor told me the primary results showed cancer in my throat and the base of my tongue. They had a lab in the building that had already begun to examine the sample. They would know for sure in a few days, and I should make an appointment to return.

At my next appointment he confirmed that the tumors in my throat were cancerous. In order to begin treatment, they needed to be sure what they were dealing with. He was convinced there was cancer in some lymph nodes on the right side of my neck as well. He also was fairly sure it was in my thyroid. He said he could feel something on the right side of my throat, so he ordered a CT scan of my neck. I believed that the results of this scan would determine whether my treatment would be radiation alone or radiation and chemotherapy. He did not recommend surgery since it would mean the removal of a large part of my tongue and possibly cutting out a piece of my throat.

CHAPTER 3
MY CRISIS OF FAITH

W
HATEVER YOUR VALUES and beliefs are about yourself and the world around you, don't be surprised if these are challenged during your experience with cancer and treatment. For me, many of my values and beliefs centered around Buddhist philosophy and practice, which I had studied and practiced for the past eight years or so.

One of the primary teachings of Buddhist philosophy is that everything is impermanent. Meditating on death and impermanence is a common Buddhist practice. This is not done out of some morbid intent but rather the belief that one can only become comfortable with living when the reality of impermanence and death are accepted. By accepting that we are impermanent beings, we can begin to understand the preciousness and value of every moment. We no longer need to live in fear, for acceptance is the opposite of fear. By knowing that our time will end, we stop wasting the time we do have, and a new appreciation is formed.

For example, if you have a favorite food you eat daily or several times a day, and knew you had an unlimited supply, you would likely take it for granted. On the other hand, if you have a favorite food and knew you may never have it again, but it was in front of you at this moment, wouldn't you approach it differently? Would you take the experience of eating that food for granted? Would you appreciate it more? Yet how often do we consider this when we think about how precious and finite our life is? Even if your faith includes believing in reincarnation and/or eternal life, we still will never have this moment, this personality, or this life again. Having a strong awareness of death is not necessarily morbid. It is a gift that helps us become more present and enjoy the preciousness of each moment. It is a reminder that this life will not last forever and should not be taken for granted.

I really thought I was comfortable with death. I had contemplated it many times. I had read about it, attended teachings about it, and meditated on it. I had friends with whom I regularly talked about death. I talked to my clients about it. I had attended workshops and presentations about death. I had watched my parents deal with their deaths and was with my mother when she died. I sat with my father just after he died.

I saw my father become so fixated on trying to make my mother better (she had dementia, and he was her primary caretaker) that he couldn't enjoy the time they had left together. I saw only fear for her and for himself. I saw little, if any, acceptance of the fact that we all will die one day. My father only lived for five months after my mother died. They had been married for fifty-eight years.

I really believed I had it all figured out. Of course, I didn't want to die, but I thought I was more enlightened about death than most, especially my parents. I envisioned meeting death with a calmness and dignity I had only seen in movies.

If the topic of cancer and treatment was ever randomly discussed, I had imagined that given the option, I would never participate in chemotherapy. I was sure that the treatment was certainly worse than death. If I had ever faced cancer and the option of chemotherapy, I would decline treatment and die gracefully.

I couldn't have been more wrong about how I would react. Once I was diagnosed, my fear of death consumed me. Everything I thought I believed, how I would be, what I would think, feel, and do, was totally different than I had anticipated. I panicked. My survival instincts kicked in, and all I could think about was that I didn't want to die. I COULD NOT DIE. I had never felt so trapped, helpless, and disillusioned. I was also angry. I was angry at my circumstance, angry at my cancer, angry that my body had betrayed me, and angry at my faith.

Buddhism teaches that things that happen in life are a result of karma. An oversimplified definition of karma from the Oxford English Dictionary is "the sum of a person's actions in this and previous states of existence, viewed as deciding their fate in future existence."

Wait a second. Does this mean that somehow I caused my own cancer? I smoked only briefly in my 20's. I didn't grow up or work around chemicals or intoxicants. I exercised, ate well, was an honest person of integrity. I even made my living helping others. How could I have caused my own cancer? Was it then, under the laws of karma, the result of something that I had done in a past life? Something I can't even recall that determined my fate before I was even born? There is no fairness in that.

My belief in my own faith crumbled even more. I could not accept that I caused this to happen, that if I had only done something differently in my life (or a past life) that I would never have been diagnosed with throat cancer.

It took time after recovery to come to terms with all of this and become comfortable with a slightly different view of karma. I have returned to my practice, but I still struggle with issues of faith, meaning, purpose, randomness, and karma. More than ever, the universe does not make sense to me. I don't believe that it ever will, and my work in this life may be to accept that. As hard as it is to admit, I don't have to understand. I joke with clients sometimes saying I have spent years studying human behavior so that I may understand more, but the more I learn the less I understand. I have found this to be true with life. The more I learn, the less I understand. Maybe that is okay.

CHAPTER 4
DIAGNOSIS (PART 2)-
FURTHER DIAGNOSTIC TESTING

A FTER THE INITIAL diagnosis, further testing was needed to know more specifics. Was my cancer localized, or had it spread to any surrounding lymph nodes or any other part of my body? This process included a CT scan of my throat, a needle biopsy of my throat, a PET scan, and visits to the ENT to discuss findings.

The diagnostic phase was scary. I frequently did not understand what it all meant, and the typical answer to my questions was we needed to run another test. My mind was all over the place. One minute I thought I was going to die, and the next I thought I would be fine with minimal treatment. Waiting was difficult.

I believe that it should be standard practice to be referred to a social worker right after a cancer diagnosis is made. Better yet, a social worker should be present and available to meet during the first appointment that cancer is even mentioned. There may likely be places in the U.S. that provide this service, but during my cancer process, this did not happen in my community.

My ENT's practice, which was a group practice of about twelve physicians, had no social worker or counselor on staff.

They owned a large multi-story building. They had several billing and scheduling specialists, nurses, medical assistants, and even their own surgery center but offered nothing in terms of mental health support, not even a referral. The only group/ organization I dealt with that had mental health support of any type was the radiation oncology clinic. Oddly, I was never informed that a social worker was even on staff at this clinic. I found out by accident after I was well into my treatment phase.

CT SCAN OF THROAT

A computed tomography scan (CT Scan) was the first step in determining if the cancer in my throat was localized or had spread to other areas of my neck. Specifically, my ENT was concerned about my thyroid and the surrounding lymph nodes. The scan was painless. I was injected with a dye and laid down onto a table where a machine imaged my neck. The machine, like so many of them through this process, looked like a large doughnut. The table would move me into the opening, and the scan only lasted a few minutes.

The worst part of this test was that the person injecting the dye could not find my vein. It took her three tries. Then after she hooked up the IV, which put the dye into my body, and started me into the machine, the tube from the IV pulled out, and warm liquid was spilled all over my arm and side. Once I was reattached, the process went well.

I had read my CT scan report online since I had computer access to my health records. The CT scan report indicated there was no cancer in my lymph nodes. It also indicated there was no cancer in my thyroid. I was extremely relieved since I was hoping this meant a less severe, more curable cancer. Most importantly, I hoped it meant that I would not have to be subjected to both radiation and chemotherapy but only radiation. In my mind, I had assumed radiation alone would be an easier treatment.

When I saw my ENT to review these results, he said he disagreed with the conclusion that there was no cancer in my lymph nodes. He believed that he could feel something abnormal on the right side of my neck. He called the radiologist who had written the report and asked him to review the X-ray again. This time the radiologist agreed there were cancer cells in at least one, maybe two, lymph nodes on the side of my neck.

This is when I really began to understand that medicine is not an exact science and doctors can have differing opinions about something I assumed would be pretty clear-cut. To be sure, my ENT recommended I have a needle biopsy of my neck. I am still not clear as to why he didn't order this in the first place.

NEEDLE BIOPSY OF MY NECK

The needle biopsy was needed to make a final determination as to whether the cells in my throat, thyroid, and lymph nodes were cancerous. This information was necessary to determine the best course of treatment and used to calibrate the radiation beams that would target the cancer cells in my neck. Using several needles (cringe), this procedure would take cell samples from my neck, which would be tested for cancer. The thought of someone sticking a needle or needles into my throat was not a pleasant one.

Just before the physician began the needle biopsy procedure, he took a live X-ray of my neck, showing me where he was going to insert the needles. He was also able to see the tumors in my throat and view my thyroid gland. He showed me images of my throat and thyroid on a screen as he did this. Looking at my thyroid, he said he did not see anything that would likely be cancer. My thyroid was shaped a little differently than most, which probably was what the concern was about, but it was within normal parameters. He would biopsy it anyway, just to be sure.

This was one of those procedures where the anticipation and fear were much worse than the procedure itself. It was not painful or even uncomfortable for more than a few seconds. The only brief discomfort came from the first injection, which was lidocaine used to numb the area. The lidocaine stings a little when it goes in. After the area was numb, I felt a little pressure and sometimes an inexplicable sensation but again no pain or discomfort. The surgeon took several samples to be reviewed.

PET SCAN

A PET scan (Positron Emission Tomography Scan) is an imaging test that X-rays your entire body. PET scans are used as a diagnostic tool for different things. In my case, the images allowed the doctors to determine if there were any other areas of my body that contained cancer cells. I was injected with a radioactive dye, which helps the imaging device see inside my body.

After the injection, which was not uncomfortable unless you have a fear of needles, I sat for about twenty-five minutes to let the dye work through my body. I didn't feel anything but a desire to take a nap. I was then taken into the PET scan room, where there was a large machine with a moving table in front of a large doughnut hole opening. It looked very similar to the CT scan machine. The table was long, hard, and narrow. I was positioned on the table which then moved into the machine. There was a technician on the other side of a clear glass window who would talk to me and hear me talk back through a microphone and speaker located in the machine itself.

I was asked to hold still for various lengths of time (up to about twenty-two minutes if I recall correctly) while the machine did its work. I felt nothing from the machine. However, lying on the hard table without moving for that length of time was not comfortable, and my back became stiff.

If you are claustrophobic, this can be difficult. It is important to tell the technician this since sometimes they don't ask. Even though I am not claustrophobic, I had a great deal of anxiety about the process and took anti-anxiety medication before I arrived for my test.

THE FINAL DIAGNOSIS AND TREATMENT RECOMMENDATION

To summarize what has happened so far, I saw my physician in July of 2017 when I first mentioned my sore throat. Between then and my official diagnosis at the end of August, I had the following procedures:

- Thyroid X-ray
- X-ray of my esophagus
- Fiberoptic laryngoscopy (where an ear, nose and throat specialist inserted a camera up my nose to see my throat)
- Throat biopsy (where a piece of the tumor was cut away and the sample sent to a lab for examination)
- CT scan of my throat
- Needle biopsy where several needles were stuck into my throat and samples of tissue were taken from lymph nodes and thyroid and sent to the lab for examination
- PET scan

None of these procedures were particularly enjoyable, but they were not awful either. I realized that in most cases the anxiety and fear were worse than the actual experience. Modern medicine has come a long way at managing discomfort.

I think it was before the needle biopsy, when I was feeling really anxious about having needles stuck in my neck, that I asked my ENT for a medication that could keep me calm. I was prescribed Lorazepam, also known as Ativan, which helped throughout my treatment process tremendously.

I had never been one to take many medications. However, I found that before, during, and after treatment, medications became extremely important. For me, having them on hand, even if I didn't use them, was something that eased my mind. Knowing they were there if I needed them calmed me down. And I did find that I used many of them throughout the process.

After receiving final confirmation that I had cancerous tumors in my throat, and the cancer had spread to at least one, possibly two lymph nodes on the side of my neck, and my thyroid was unaffected—I was referred to a radiation oncologist and a medical oncologist. I had no idea what the difference was or what this meant. I would not see the ENT again until four months after my treatment was completed.

I was never clear if my cancer was stage III or stage IV. Almost all of the throat cancer survivors I spoke with had been diagnosed with stage III or stage IV cancer. Regardless of which stage it was, my cancer was advanced and had spread to at least one lymph node. At first, this terrified me. I remember hearing stories of advanced cancer being a death sentence. However, the staging process of cancer doesn't mean what it used to or what I had believed it meant. The severity is not only determined by stage but also where the cancer is located. I was told by my ENT that there was good news and bad news (I really hate when doctors say this). The bad news was that I had an extremely fast growing, aggressive type of cancer. This is likely why most throat cancers, by the time they are seen, are already stage IV. The good news was that it was "highly treatable and had positive outcomes." He said something like that without using the word "curable," which doctors never do. In doctor speak, he said that I was likely going to be okay.

Something worth noting here. Physicians have their own language, which is different from mine. I found myself waiting to be reassured about being cured, but they don't speak that way. They always seemed cautious in their prognosis and their interpretation. They are trained to look for and deal with disease. This is their strength. Diagnosis and treatment issues appear to be in their comfort zone. Prevention, recovery, and particularly reassurance, not so much. Again, there are some exceptions to this, but in my experience, this was mostly the case. Once I understood this, I could relax a little knowing that a clear prognosis was not something I would ever get from a physician. For this type of information, I would rely on other cancer survivors, always realizing that my experience could differ.

I was talking to a friend who has several different cancers throughout her body and has been in treatment for a few years. When talking about her experience with doctors and some other medical professionals, her opinion was that "doctors need to take off their white coats and start seeing their patients as more human." I would agree with this. If the medical community saw patients as if they were family members, for example, receiving medical care would likely be a different experience.

CHAPTER 5
PREPARATION FOR TREATMENT

AFTER I WAS diagnosed with throat cancer and learned the details regarding where it had spread and how severe it was, preparation for treatment began. Preparation for treatment was intense. There were further evaluations, testing, and procedures that needed to be completed before treatment began.

Before my diagnosis I had felt fine except for, as I had said, a little scratchy throat. After my diagnosis, I felt like I was already in treatment. I was scared, overwhelmed, confused, angry, depressed, and anxious. My appetite went away, and I felt nauseous all the time.

Given the same circumstance, individual reactions, fears, thoughts, and concerns can vary a great deal. For me, I was extremely concerned about being nauseous and vomiting once treatment began. I really had never heard much about radiation treatment. However, I had heard things about chemotherapy, and none of them were good. I had heard about weakness, hair loss, weight loss, and the worst—nausea and vomiting.

Since my diagnosis, I couldn't stop thinking about dying or what it would be like to live through treatment, which sometimes scared me more. I still hoped that after meeting with the medical oncologist, I would be told I only needed radiation.

The following list is not necessarily inclusive and not all of these may be needed for your situation, but this is what I needed to do before I was able to start treatment. The preparation process took about a month.

- Meeting with a radiation oncologist
- Dental examination and treatment
- Port insertion (surgery)
- Feeding tube insertion (surgery)
- Meetings with a medical oncologist
- Chemotherapy educational workshop
- Radiation mask fitting and testing
- Meeting with a dietitian
- Meeting with a speech therapist

THE RADIATION ONCOLOGIST

The radiation oncologist was the first doctor I saw after the ENT gave me my official diagnosis. The radiation oncologist was the physician in charge of the radiation that would target the area of my throat that contained the cancer. I learned that in order to make sure all the cancer was radiated, the target area would be all areas of my neck and jaw.

During my first appointment, the radiation oncologist rambled on for what seemed like hours about the structure of my throat, the possible nasty side effects of the treatment, and the things that had to happen before the treatment began. An invisible, painless beam (or beams) of radiation would be aimed at the tumors and lymph nodes for a period of about five minutes per day for thirty-three consecutive days, excluding weekends. The whole process would take about twenty minutes. I would experience a "cumulative" effect and likely damage to my saliva glands and taste buds. It would cause throat pain and impede my ability to swallow. In some instances, it could weaken my jaw, cause root damage to my teeth, cause sores in my mouth and on my tongue...and he went on. I would experience the side effects after about two weeks of treatment. The skin on my neck would react as if it had a bad sunburn and turn red, become scaly, and slough off. He went on to say that as I began to recover, I would start producing sticky saliva but would not be able to swallow, so I would be spitting into a rag or a cup for a while. Since I would have such difficulty swallowing, I would likely need a feeding tube, which he preferred to have put in before treatment started.

Somewhere in his well-practiced speech, I heard something about a ninety percent cure rate for this type of cancer though I don't believe any doctor I saw ever used the word "cure". He used terms like "positive treatment outcomes" and "five-year survival rates". Someone decided that if you survive five years cancer free after treatment, that you are considered "cured" though again they don't use that word. They say you are in "sustained remission".

I felt totally overwhelmed. If I was to rate the performance of my radiation oncologist, I would give him a D+ for his ability to connect with a patient or be empathetic. I walked out of his office depressed, angry, and terrified. In hindsight, I shouldn't have expected him to have a good bedside manner though it would have been helpful. I assume (since I survived) that he was technically skilled, which is what I would want in a radiation oncologist. His bedside manner was not particularly good, but I didn't need a radiation oncologist who could take care of my feelings. I needed one who had the technical skills to make sure that the radiation beam destroyed the cancerous tumors while doing as little damage as possible to the other structures in my throat and mouth. I would find my emotional support elsewhere.

Preparing for treatment meant several meetings with this doctor to talk about and verify completion of the steps necessary to be ready to begin radiation treatment. I was amazed at the successful coordination between providers given everything that had to happen before treatment could begin.

THE MEDICAL ONCOLOGIST

The next major medical appointment was with a medical oncologist. This was the doctor who would decide if chemotherapy was recommended and, if so, would oversee all treatment.

I loved my medical oncologist. She was one of my saving graces throughout the whole process. She was the only professional who told me I would be okay, and at one point she even used the word "cure". She was kind, knowledgeable, empathetic, pragmatic, and honest.

She worked many hours and saw many patients, yet she took her time with me, was patient and reassuring, didn't sit behind a computer, or take many notes during our meeting. She seemed to remember everything, and I don't know how she did it.

My understanding of chemotherapy is that you sit in a chair and a nurse injects poison into your veins, or you take pills that are poison or receive both injections and pills. The poison kills cancer cells, also kills healthy cells, and can cause many different side effects. The medical oncologist's job is to pick the right poison for your particular type of cancer and make sure you get enough of it to kill the cancer without killing the patient. I still hoped that I would not need chemotherapy.

A few days after my first appointment with the medical oncologist, I received a call from her front desk person who said the doctor wanted me to come in for an educational workshop on chemotherapy. "What? Why?" I asked. "No one has told me anything. Does this mean I need chemotherapy?".

The woman on the phone paused, stuttered, and then said, "Let me have the doctor call you." Within the hour the medical oncologist called me and apologized for the way this was handled. She said that she had reviewed the X-rays and the needle biopsy results and had spoken to the radiation oncologist. She said that they agreed the best chance for me would be to participate concurrently in radiation treatment and chemotherapy. She would support whatever I decided, if I decided I only wanted radiation, but her recommendation was for both. She said that because I was young and in good shape (thank you for saying I was young), they wanted to treat my cancer aggressively to give me the best chance of remission and it not coming back. By "aggressively", she meant with both radiation and chemotherapy.

I realized that either treatment on its own presented several challenges but doing them concurrently would be especially difficult. However, I did know from doing some of my own research, that for my type of cancer I would have a better than ninety percent chance of a cure if I completed both treatments. In fact, she told me that in her entire career, she had only seen one recurrence and that was a man who was much older than me, had smoked for thirty years, and continued to smoke before, during, and after treatment. I decided if I was going to go through treatment, I would have both radiation and chemotherapy. I scheduled myself for the chemotherapy educational workshop.

TAKING A BREAK

Some good friends were leaving for a week vacation to Canmore, Canada. I looked it up online and saw how beautiful it was. I thought about how long it might be before I would be physically able to go to a place like this or if I would ever be able to see a place like this again. I was talking to my friend just before she and her husband left and jokingly said that my wife and I would be "crashing" their vacation. She took my joke seriously and told me she and her husband were all for it. So, at the last minute we postponed all of my appointments another week and headed to Canada for a vacation. I made the decision I was going to shut down my practice before our vacation and not worry about it until after treatment.

I was lucky I had good health insurance and did not have to work during treatment. I understand that many are not so lucky. We do what we have to do. I know there would have been no way I could have worked during treatment. Yet I know many people who do. The ability to work, like so many issues related to cancer and treatment, will vary from person to person.

Canmore and the surrounding area are amazing places to visit. Snow covered mountains, clear rivers, turquoise lakes, and glaciers, were all part of the beauty and serenity. The food was great, and the people were warm and friendly. Being in Canmore, the thought of cancer and treatment seemed far away. I still only experienced my cancer as a scratchy throat which didn't bother me much.

It was hard to remember that I had cancer. Aside from not having much of an appetite (probably a bit in shock still), I felt fine. I was able to physically do anything I wanted during the vacation. I experienced no physical limitations at all. On vacation, we hiked, ate, explored, and had a great time.

This turned out to be very important for me to do before starting treatment. Having a little distance on what had been happening, and not spending my days obsessed with my medical condition, was a huge relief.

After our week in Canmore, I returned to the reality of preparing for treatment. There were still many things that needed to be done. Memories of Canmore helped me go to my happy place more than once when things felt bleak.

DENTAL EXAMINATION AND TREATMENT

Because the radiation treatment had the potential of affecting my teeth, gums, roots, and jawbone, it was necessary to have a dental examination and any recommended dental work completed before I could begin treatment. For me this meant an exam and a cavity that needed to be filled. For others this could be a big thing. I have heard stories of people who had put off going to the dentist for years and now had to have work completed that should have been done a long time ago. My radiation oncologist asked for a letter signed by my dentist, stating I was in good dental health, before moving forward with treatment.

PORT INSERTION

When I agreed with the recommendation for chemo-therapy, the medical oncologist recommended I have a port put into my chest. At the time, I had no idea what this was.

A port is a small disc made of plastic or metal (mine was metal) inserted under the skin. A thin tube, or catheter (also under the skin), connects the port to a large vein. The port was inserted into my chest just below my clavicle on my right side. It stayed in during and after treatment, until it was determined that my cancer was gone. It is used with a special needle in order to provide easy access for the chemotherapy drugs. It can also be used for other injections or blood draws.

I did not want a port. The thought of this metal thing living in my chest did not thrill me. If I had chosen to not have the port, each chemotherapy session would require an IV needle, which would be injected and fixed into my hand or arm. Not having a port meant that a nurse would have to find a good vein before each treatment, and I would have to be careful having an IV in me for eight-hour chemotherapy sessions. (I was up and down a lot during the session, which I will explain later). Also, the IV would have caused bruising around the insertion point.

I chose to have the port, and I am glad I did. It was easy to use, secure, and eventually I barely felt the needle insertion. The downside was it left two distinct scars on my chest— one from when it went in and one from when it came out. It also protruded a bit from under my skin and could easily be bumped, which hurt. Some people have trouble with seat belts rubbing against the port and causing discomfort, but I never had this issue.

A surgeon inserted the port. I was not put to sleep, but rather he numbed the area on my chest with an injection of lidocaine. The lidocaine stung a little, but then the area went numb quickly. He put a light drape over my face, made an incision in my chest, and inserted the port. I am guessing by the size of the scar that the incision was no more than a few inches. I felt some pressure and some tugging but nothing else. After the port was placed, the incision was glued shut. It was sore for maybe a week or so, and I had to be careful when showering.

If you do have a port inserted, it is a good idea to allow the skin around it to heal for at least a few weeks before it is used.

If I recall correctly, I had my port placed three days before my first chemotherapy treatment. My skin around it was still raw and sore. Before the needle was inserted, I had iced the area and put topical numbing cream on it. Even so, when that needle was inserted into my port, I experienced some of the worst pain I had felt during my whole cancer process. I imagined that is what it felt like to be stabbed. I should have had the port inserted earlier so the area around it could have healed.

Once my skin around the port area healed, I barely felt the needle at all and did not have to use any ice or numbing cream prior to a needle being inserted. If you do experience any discomfort, ice and numbing cream should be available. The numbing cream I used was by prescription, obtained from my medical oncologist, and applied about a half an hour before the port was used. The nurses at the medical oncology center were always happy to provide me with ice to use for a few minutes before the needle was inserted into the port.

FEEDING TUBE INSERTION

Most people imagine a feeding tube going down the throat and staying there. This is not correct for feeding tubes for throat cancer treatment. This tube, also referred to as a PEG tube or G tube, was placed in my stomach through my abdomen. The feeding tube insertion procedure may vary depending on what type of tube is being inserted. I was put to sleep for my procedure. My tube had to be first inserted down my throat and then through my stomach and out my abdomen. It protruded about six inches from my abdomen. Nothing remained in my throat. The hole in my abdomen called the stoma, where the tube came out, was about a quarter inch in diameter. Feeding through the tube meant that whatever went in went directly into my stomach. The need for the tube began when it became difficult to swallow and food and water began to taste really

51

bad. This was about two weeks after my first radiation treatment and a week after my first chemotherapy treatment.

I had trouble with my feeding tube from day one, which I discuss in detail later. Most people don't have the problems I had, but the area around the tube is likely to be sore for a while. It is not something you can lie on, and it will hurt when it is bumped. You are living with a hole in your abdomen, which will be tender for a while. If you have a tube like I did, it needs to be secured (e.g. taped to your stomach) under your clothes so it doesn't accidentally pull. At first, I was self-conscious about people seeing it under my shirt, but at some point, I stopped caring.

There was the availability of something called a "MIC-KEY tube" which, instead of sticking out, is almost flush with your skin. I don't know how decisions are made as to what type of tube is used when (seems random to me), but it is something that can be requested. Though I could have changed to this type of tube, I chose not to. My decision was based on the amount of pain and irritation I had and continued to have around the stoma area. I did not want to risk infecting it or experiencing further irritation by changing my tube. Having to have my current tube pulled out and a new one put in when the stoma was already somewhat inflamed, would have caused me more grief.

CHEMOTHERAPY EDUCATIONAL WORKSHOP

Part of preparing for chemotherapy included meeting with an oncology nurse, who explained the chemotherapy process, provided written information, presented me with a pile of forms that needed to be signed, discussed possible side effects, and answered questions. I should have walked out of the chemotherapy educational session after the first five minutes.

I sat in a small room with my wife and an oncology nurse, who appeared bored and burned out, barely making eye contact with me and yawning much of the time. She started reading from a mound of paperwork, which covered everything from my rights to the names of the drugs they would put in me, to the possible side effects of treatment. I was anxious before attending this meeting, and her manor made me more anxious. I asked her twice to stop reading the list of possible side effects. It was too much for me to hear. But she said it was required and kept going. I should have left.

At one point, after reading countless unpleasant possible side effects that I could experience, she said something to the effect of "we are not trying to torture you." I responded by saying it sounded like they were. She paused, looked at me, and said in a snippy tone, "Well, that is your perception," and continued with her reading. After she was finished, I left feeling hopeless.

As it turned out, many of the things on her list (and I swear there must be 100 possible side effects from chemotherapy drugs), I never experienced. There is no way to predict what side effects will occur and how someone will experience them.

The one small piece of good news I took from this was that given the type of chemotherapy drug I would receive, hair loss, which includes losing eyebrows and eyelashes, was extremely unlikely. I would be allowed to keep what little hair on my head I had left, most of which I had lost all on my own.

There was no excuse for how that educational material was presented. I think it was then, or soon after, that I discussed a new strategy with my wife. Though hearing all the possible bad news was hard for her, she handled it better than I did. We agreed it was not good for me to be presented with a great deal of negative information. She would be the one who would receive whatever information was required to be given. There were folders and folders of written information in addition to the verbal information I received at every medical appointment. She would be in charge of keeping and reading these as well. I got to a point where I would not read any of the written handouts anymore, and I tuned out most of the verbal information unless there was something specific I wanted to know. She was also tasked with deciding if I needed to know something or not. I could ask specific questions if I needed to, but she was the one who took notes and carried around the volumes of written material every medical provider at every appointment handed out. This was one of the many things she did for me that I so much appreciated. I could focus on whatever was happening in the moment, keep up with the things I was asked to do daily during treatment, and try to keep my mind from spinning.

As it turned out, the nurse who had conducted my educational workshop was assigned to me as my oncology nurse for one of my chemotherapy sessions. I was assigned a different nurse for the day for each session. At first, I considered asking for a different nurse but then decided I would give her some feedback about my perception of her workshop as nicely as I could. I did my best to be kind about how I gave her feedback, and she was receptive to it. She apologized to me and shared she was pretty burned out. I had not thought much about how hard of a job it must be to work with cancer patients all day long. Nor had I realized that the professionals don't have much support for the emotional toll their job must have on them. More about this in the section about compassion.

THE MASK

My radiation oncologist kept talking to me about being fitted for a mask prior to the start of radiation treatment. There was so much information coming at me that I had not given this any thought until I had an appointment specifically to be fitted for a mask, which I still didn't quite understand.

Targeting radiation beams to the throat can be tricky. I had no knowledge of the anatomy of my mouth and throat and was surprised at how many structures there are and what they do. Pointing beams of radiation at these structures has the potential of damaging them. It is inevitable that there will be some damage. Some of the damage will repair itself given time. Some will not.

There were several considerations in figuring out how to aim the radiation beams. How this was all determined and calculated is way beyond my comprehension. The beams needed to be powerful, accurate, and broad enough to kill the cancer cells where they currently lived and nearby where they might likely live. This had to be balanced with doing as little damage to the existing structures of my throat and mouth as possible. For throat cancer, this meant trying to do minimal damage to my taste buds, saliva glands, thyroid gland, vocal cords, and many other complex parts of my throat and mouth that help me breath, eat, swallow, and so on. This seemed like a tall order.

If this was not hard enough, the success of this treatment and the minimization of long-term damage also depended on the patient not moving during this treatment. Moving would redirect the beam. These beams are calibrated to be extremely accurate, and it could be damaging if they did not hit the right targets.

Hence the problem. How do you keep a human being from moving during a fifteen- to twenty-minute process? The solution? Bolt them to a table.

Two men greeted me at my mask fitting appointment. The man in the shorts and a T-shirt introduced himself as a technician who would be making the mask. The other, who wore slacks, a dress shirt, and a tie was introduced as the consultant. His job was to pace around with his hand on his chin saying, "Hmmmm," while the technician did the work.

I was asked to lie face up on a hard table and relax, a bit of a contradiction. The technician explained they would make a mask that would fit over my face, head, and neck, going slightly down my chest. The back of the mask would fit flush against the table and then be attached to it. This mask would be used during radiation treatments as a way of keeping me immobile.

If the idea of this is making you anxious, you are not alone. For me, anxiety at every step was part of my process. I came to know it intimately and did ultimately develop some strategies, including taking medications, to deal with it.

The technician said I would feel a warm plastic mesh being positioned over my face (you can look online for radiation mask making and find many videos of this procedure). The mesh is first heated, which makes it pliable. The mesh is full of holes, so breathing was not an issue. After laying it over my face, they lock it down to the table. This forces the mask to contour to my face, head, and neck. I was asked to lie still for several minutes while the mask hardened.

Once hardened, it retained the shape of my face, head, neck, and shoulders. Each mask may be longer or shorter than mine (my mask covered part of my chest, but some masks won't go down past the chin). I really don't know how this decision is made about what size the mask needs to be, but that is for the radiation oncologist and technicians to figure out.

The mask was tight, not painful but confining. I remember thinking I needed to close my eyes before they put it on me again because my eyelashes were touching the inside of the mask making it hard for me to close my eyes while the mask was on me. They also fitted me with a mouth guard, like what a boxer wears, that I would need to keep in my mouth while the mask was on. This kept my tongue and jaw from moving during radiation treatment. It also kept me from being able to talk.

This process of being locked down to a table with a mask on is hard for most people. You may recall that I took an anti-anxiety pill before having my neck needle biopsy. I took an anti-anxiety pill before most of my radiation treatments.

In time, it became much easier to deal with the radiation procedure. Toward the end of my radiation treatments, I could even nap during the process.

In terms of advocating for yourself, dealing with the mask and the process of being locked down to a table is one time you might need to speak up. If the thought of the mask causes anxiety, you can ask for practice sessions. Maybe at first you lie on the table and try to relax. Once relaxed, the mask is placed over you without being locked down. After you become used to this, the mask may be locked down for a few seconds and then released. Gradually you spend more time being locked down until you get used to it. In psychology we call this step-by-step approach while learning to relax at each step, systematic desensitization. It is a highly effective intervention that has been around since the 1940s, and yet it is unlikely that anyone will suggest a process like this to you. As I will repeat many times, the majority of medical procedures do not take into account psychological factors. The medical community is there to deal with your cancer, not your anxiety.

Throughout the process of my cancer diagnosis and preparation, I have used the word "trapped". I felt trapped by my diagnosis. I felt trapped by my options. I felt trapped when I didn't want to listen to the possible side effects of chemotherapy. And now, literally, I was being physically trapped by having a mask put over me and locked to the table I was lying on, which in effect, immobilized me.

MEETING WITH THE DIETICIAN

I did not have good experiences with the dieticians whom I worked with during my cancer process. They seemed overworked, short on time, and neglected to impart important information that I later had to discover on my own. This information would have saved me a great deal of discomfort (see the section on my feeding tube for the details).

The dietitian's job, as I understood, was to make sure I took in enough calories and nutrients throughout treatment and into recovery. This also included making sure I had enough water each day. When I was unable to eat and had to use a feeding tube, the dietitian was supposed to work with me on finding the best feeding tube formula and be there to deal with any concerns that I had. This didn't happen, which I discuss later in more detail.

CHAPTER 6
TREATMENT

THE TRANSITION FROM preparation to treatment was marked for me by my first radiation session on October 16, 2017. My treatment consisted of thirty-three days of consecutive radiation to my throat (except weekends) and six rounds of chemotherapy (one full day per week for six consecutive weeks). It also eventually included two- to three-hour daily hydration sessions, six days a week, for a period of about two months.

Overall, the team of professionals whom I worked with was great at addressing my medical needs. The coordination it took between offices was amazing and went smoothly. Many times during the cancer process, I felt as if I was receiving too much attention.

The infusion group, who supplied my feeding tube, formula, and supplies, called me regularly. The check-ins were appreciated, but I was asked many standard and sometimes annoying questions, like "How many boxes of formula did I use a day? How many ounces of water did I ingest a day? Can I rate my pain on a scale of one to ten?" I got tired of the questions and often couldn't answer them. If I answered in a way that concerned them, like not having enough ounces of water per day, I received a lecture.

I was constantly lectured about not taking in enough feeding formula or water and about losing weight. At some point I told the person to stop lecturing me—that I wasn't going listen to any more lectures and that many of the questions I couldn't answer.

In hindsight, I realized there were two reasons for all of the questions. First, they were required to document my progress and were monitoring what was happening with me. Second, I learned the hard way that during the cancer process a medical problem can develop quickly, and some did. The questions and the lectures were an attempt to prevent serious issues.

MY DAILY SCHEDULE

People asked me what I did with my time off during treatment and recovery. Some people actually asked me to do some projects for them during this time, "in case I was bored." I didn't start a single project.

I wasn't feeling particularly motivated to do much. Some of the hobbies I had enjoyed prior to the start of the cancer process, I no longer had an interest in. Luckily, the interest returned after treatment was completed. There would have not been much time to do anything anyway. A fact that surprised me.

A typical schedule for me during treatment included:

- Twenty hours per day using my feeding tube pump where I had to constantly check formula levels, add formula, and change out the tape and tubing as needed.
- Changing gauze and tape around my stoma—the hole in my stomach where the feeding tube went in—and cleaning the area at least twice daily.
- Completing several swallowing exercises each day that my speech therapist gave me.

- Making sure I stayed on whatever my drug regimens happened to be, which changed depending on my needs. It was important to stay ahead of any pain or nausea that might occur.
- Attending daily radiation appointments, Monday – Friday, for about an hour to an hour and a half each day, which included travel, wait time, and the actual procedure, for thirty-three consecutive days (excluding weekends).
- Attending daily hydration appointments for two to three hours per day, six days per week. I attended these for about two months.
- Attending chemotherapy one day per week, eight hours each time, for six weeks (I still had to go have radiation treatments on these days as well).
- Attending weekly appointments with the radiation oncologist.
- Attending weekly appointments with the medical oncologist.
- Attending weekly appointments with the social worker.
- Completing weekly blood work to make sure my body continued to function.
- Attending biweekly appointments with my speech therapist.
- Using dental trays for a half an hour daily for fluoride treatments.
- Inspecting my mouth daily for any sores or changes.

During my treatment I also experienced a visit to urgent care, a night in the emergency room, and a three-day/two-night stay in the hospital. Given my schedule, you will see there were not enough hours in the day. And I was supposed to rest as well.

RADIATION

Each of my thirty-three radiation treatments began with a technician walking me into a room that contained the radiation machine. I took off my shirt and laid face up on a long narrow table. A technician put a blanket over me (often a heated one which felt good) and handed me the mouth guard that I put in my mouth and bit down on. The mask that covered my head, face, neck, and shoulders was stored on site and was then put over me and locked to the table. The technician asked if I was ready, and I grunted, not being able to talk with the mouth guard in place. The table then moved me into the opening of the tube.

Each machine that delivers the radiation beams can look different. A quick search online shows some machines that are totally open while others, as in my case, looked like I was being pulled into a large doughnut. Luckily, I am not claustrophobic, but this didn't mean this was not challenging. Again, if you are going to be in an enclosed space for your treatment, you can request practice sessions and take very small steps until you can spend the amount of time needed in your mask and in the "tunnel".

Once I was settled, the technician would go to another room where I was watched on camera. For the first five or so minutes, the machine made a humming sound, but no radiation was being used. My understanding is that this was a time when the machine calibrated where the beams would target. Somehow, they were able to figure out how to send the beams to exactly the same areas each time, and it took a few minutes for them to verify this.

The next few minutes were quiet as the radiation oncologist and/or radiological technicians viewed the calibration and determined that it was accurate. When we were a "go", the machine turned on again, and I heard the distinct sound it made as the radiation beams were applied. It sounded a little like a Native American rain stick being turned over. It was not loud, just distinct. There were no flashes of light, and I could not feel the radiation. This went on for about five minutes as well. When it stopped, a technician came back into the room, and the table slid out of the tunnel. The technician unlocked the mask, removed the mouth guard, and helped me sit up. The whole process, from being locked to the table to being unlocked, took fifteen to twenty minutes.

The process took some getting used to. The good news is you do not feel the radiation beams, and there is no pain during the process. At first the mask was extremely tight, to the point where my eyelashes were pressed against it on the inside and opening and closing my eyes was difficult. By the end of my radiation treatments, I had lost so much weight that I was able to move around freely under the mask. However, I didn't dare, afraid that if I did, I would misdirect the radiation beams.

I became accustomed to this process. I became familiar with the sounds of the machine and could predict how much longer each stage of the process would take. Instead of fifteen to twenty minutes, I only had to wait five minutes for calibration, then five minutes for approval, and then five minutes for radiation. Breaking it down into increments was helpful for me.

I also visualized and typically kept my eyes closed through the whole process. I went to my happy places—the beach, the woods. Toward the end of radiation treatments, I napped through the process.

SOME SUGGESTIONS FOR DEALING WITH RADIATION TREATMENTS INCLUDE:

1. Consider taking anti-anxiety medication before the mask making process and even before each radiation treatment.

2. Concentrate and focus on your breathing. Practice closing your eyes and focusing on your breath.

3. There are professionals who specialize in helping with claustrophobia. Seek one out if needed.

4. Go to your happy place. I spent a lot of time on a beach in Mexico in my head while I received radiation therapy.

5. Distract yourself. Count the holes in the ceiling, make up nonsense words and definitions that start with each letter of the alphabet, review your happiest childhood memories, create your ideal fantasy sports team. Use your mind to distract yourself from what is happening.

6. Explore what is happening (this is the opposite of distraction). Tune into every sensation. What do you hear? What do you see? Smell? Feel? What is it like to feel anxiety, for example? What does it look like? Does it have shape, color, or mass? Use your mind as if you were a detective watching and analyzing what you are going through.

7. Visualize the radiation beams entering the cancer cells and destroying them. Picture the beams in detail, seeing the size, color, and intensity. Visualize the cancer cells, what they look like and what they act like. Watch as each beam pulverizes the cancer cells. You can picture it

as a video game. Imagine yourself feeling stronger and stronger with the destruction of each cell.

8. At least one technician will be watching you during every treatment. Work out a signal that means you need to get out ASAP (remember with the bite guard in you can't talk). This will not be unfamiliar to them, and knowing you have a way out if needed can be helpful. Once you give the signal, they can turn off the machine, and get you out and unlocked from the table in seconds.

CHEMOTHERAPY

My wife and I learned quickly to pack a "go bag" for chemotherapy. This was in addition to carrying my feeding pump and the backpack for it, which I was using by my second chemotherapy session. The bag included music headphones, my computer tablet, medications, my feeding tube supplies (tape, formula, etc.), numbing cream for my port, a wool cap, snacks when I was able to eat them, and an electric blanket.

Buying an electric blanket was one of those little things that made life much more comfortable during treatment. I was cold much of the time, and I used the blanket during chemotherapy and frequently at home. I would highly recommend buying an electric blanket. It is not uncommon for cancer treatment to throw off your body temperature.

The chemotherapy center was a large building complete with doctor's offices, an infusion center, a laboratory for blood draws and testing, and a separate waiting room. A large, almost circular desk with at least six different individuals sitting in the round behind it was what I first saw when I walked in. I checked in and checked out at this desk.

After I was called into the infusion room, I was directed to a large, reclining chair. The chairs were spaced a few feet apart, and a curtain could be drawn around the chair if desired. The chairs were comfortable, and each individual area had its own television. In a central area of the room, a table had pitchers of water, assorted snacks, and juices.

At any given time, the infusion room must have had fifteen to twenty patients receiving chemotherapy drugs and at least half a dozen oncology nurses. I was assigned a nurse for each chemotherapy treatment. My treatment was once a week for about eight hours for six weeks. On the days I had chemotherapy, I had to attend my radiation appointment before my chemotherapy session.

After I was in the reclining chair, the nurse started an IV drip using my port. Of the eight hours I was in the infusion room, I had something being pumped into me the whole time. However, I received my chemotherapy drug, Cisplatin, for only about forty minutes of this time. I was given fluids for hydration for the first few hours, and then I was given Lasix (Furosemide), which is a diuretic. This would make me urinate, which was the goal, to flush out my kidneys and make sure they were working okay.

The Lasix became a bit of a joke for me. I could sit for the first several hours of my treatment while I was being hydrated and maybe go to the bathroom once. Once the Lasix was used, I was up every ten minutes, dragging my IV stand and bags of fluids with me. My personal record was having to urinate fifteen times within a few hours. I kept asking if I would win something for this, but I never received an answer. Humor in a room full of cancer patients was often not well received.

After the Lasix, came the chemotherapy drug, Cisplatin. I never realized how many different chemotherapy drugs there were. Each drug targets different cancers and has its own specific side effects. Cisplatin was the drug of choice for my type of cancer and is generally used for throat cancer treatment. I remember wondering what it would feel like to have the Cisplatin injected into my system. I never felt anything during or immediately after the infusion.

Once the Cisplatin was in my system, I received more hydration. After about eight hours of sitting in the chemo chair, I was sent home. I didn't start to feel bad until about the third day after each chemotherapy treatment. For me that meant nausea, tiredness, and some other issues that I talk more about in the section on side effects.

You will literally be toxic for a few days after a chemotherapy treatment. My wife and I were told that for three days after each chemotherapy treatment there should be no exchange of body fluids. If possible, we should use different toilets, not share any utensils, and not drink out of the same container. It was an odd feeling to know that I was poisonous, and yet somehow being full of poison was supposed to save my life.

SPEECH THERAPY

I had met with a speech therapist briefly before treatment began. It was another situation where I was receiving so much information I didn't really hear or understand much of it, including why I would even need to see a speech therapist.

During the treatment of throat cancer (most commonly due to the radiation treatment), swallowing can become a problem. Depending on where exactly the cancer is located in the throat and if there has to be any surgery (and the location of the surgery), speaking clearly can become an issue as well—hence, the speech therapist.

Much of what was done was preventive. She wanted me to do mouth and breathing exercises daily to help prevent problems that may occur. She monitored my ability to speak, the strength of my mouth, throat, and tongue muscles, and my ability to swallow. If any of these things became problematic, she could introduce techniques (and sometime apparatus) that I could use for rehabilitation.

She assigned me exercises to do daily, which included chewing on what I am convinced was really a dog chew toy. I was to do jaw and tongue exercises as well as vocal exercises. I was given a spirometer, a device with a tube attached to it, that I would inhale into. Inhaling into the tube moved a floating indicator located inside the device. This measured my lungs' ability to take in air and could be used to train my lungs to take in more. These exercises took five to ten minutes per day, and then I met with the speech therapist weekly or biweekly to review my progress and discuss questions.

I was very lucky that I was always able to swallow without any obstructions. Though painful, it was always possible. My speech was not impacted at all, and the muscles in my mouth, throat, and tongue were strong. The whole speech therapy experience was more precautionary than anything else, and I was quickly discharged from having to attend appointments soon after treatment ended.

I really liked my speech therapist. She was positive and kind, and I found these things to be so incredibly valuable. This was especially true when I was experiencing the worst side effects from treatment and feeling sorry for myself. It was always a positive experience to see her. This was because of who she was, how she connected with people, and how kind she was. It had nothing to do with any medical treatment I received from her.

HYDRATION

I don't recall if I had completed one or two chemotherapy sessions, but I had become severely dehydrated—partly due to the chemotherapy drug and partly due to not taking in enough daily fluid through my feeding tube. This landed me in the emergency room where I was rehydrated and then instructed to attend daily hydration sessions, which included weekends. For the next few months, I spent two to three hours per day, six days per week (not on my chemo days since I was hydrated during the chemotherapy), sitting in an infusion room receiving hydration. This was in addition to my daily radiation sessions, my weekly day long chemotherapy session, and all my other appointments.

These hydration sessions were extremely important, and I never understood why this was not a standard part of treatment. Being dehydrated made me feel really bad, which I had attributed to being part of the side effects of treatment that I couldn't do anything about. This was not true. Receiving hydration daily helped a great deal.

MEDICATIONS

You will likely be given or offered a variety of medications throughout treatment. You will have to decide what works for you. Some people do not like taking medication. I was one of those people, and this changed for me during treatment. The most important medications for me during the cancer process were medications for anxiety, pain, and nausea. The process would have been much worse for me without these.

I also realized that taking these medications before a problem developed, before I started feeling nauseous, or before I started feeling anxiety, helped. Knowing that I had medications available to me, meaning that I had the prescriptions filled and within reach, was a comfort even if I didn't need them.

I found that most of the doctors I worked with had no problem dispensing medications. However, there was one physician I dealt with who was reluctant to give me medication until he felt I absolutely needed it, meaning he was not comfortable writing me a prescription to have on hand if needed. I learned early on that rather than fighting him on this, I went to one of my many other doctors and got what I needed. In fact, most of the time I got much more than I needed, and I had many bottles of medication left over when I concluded my treatment.

I am sure the pain medication helped, but in general the pain was much more tolerable than I had feared. It hurt when I swallowed, but due to using a feeding tube and the fact that the radiation dried up my saliva, I had little need to swallow, so I felt little pain.

Below is a list of the medications I was on and what they were for during my cancer process. This does not include the chemotherapy drug.

- Trazodone – sleep
- Ambien – sleep
- Melatonin – sleep
- Hydrocodone (Norco) – pain
- Fentanyl – pain
- Omeprazole – acid reducer
- Ondansetron – nausea
- Diazepam – anxiety
- Hydroxyzine – anxiety
- Lorazepam – anxiety
- Fluconazole – oral thrush
- Nystatin – oral thrush

OTHER SIDE EFFECTS AND ANNOYANCES DURING TREATMENT

I wish there was a clear road map so that each cancer patient could know exactly what side effects would occur. Unfortunately, this is not the case. I can only speak about the side effects and annoyances I experienced during my process. As the facilitator of my head and neck cancer support group says, "Your mileage may vary."

FOOD AND DRINK

For almost everyone who goes through mouth or throat cancer treatment, eating and nutrition are big issues. For most who receive treatment for head and neck cancer, a feeding tube is necessary. This is due mostly to the swallowing difficulty caused by the radiation, most of which eventually heals.

The other major contributing factor to not eating is that the taste of everything changes for the worse. Food tasted so bad that even if I could have eaten, I would not have—hence, the need for the feeding tube.

I remember a specific moment in the middle of my treatment when I became aware of how much I wanted to regain my ability to drink a big glass of water again. This was a good reminder of how much I took for granted before treatment.

MOUTH AND THROAT ISSUES

Again, I want to make it clear that the side effects experienced during treatment and recovery vary greatly from individual to individual. I am sharing my personal experience which may or may not be part of your experience. The only guarantee is that there will be side effects. It is not possible to predict exactly what yours will be, the duration, or the intensity.

As radiation progressed, my throat became very sore, and it became painful to swallow. The majority of the time it felt minor, but even at its worst, I found it manageable.

For throat pain caused by the radiation, I used medications—hydrocodone and fentanyl to be exact. Hydrocodone came in pill and liquid form that could be inserted into my feeding tube. Fentanyl was a patch that I wore and was constantly absorbed into my system.

The radiation also caused my saliva to dry up, and my mouth became very dry. What I didn't understand is that not only does saliva help us with swallowing food, but it also helps protect our mouths, especially our teeth, from bacteria. Combine this lack of protection due to a dry mouth with the fact that radiation can weaken teeth, cause mouth sores, and weaken the jaw structure, and it becomes apparent that mouth care during treatment and recovery is very important.

Before treatment, my dentist made me mouth trays to be used for daily fluoride treatments. He wanted me to do two fluoride treatments each day (a half hour for each treatment) along with brushing my teeth with a prescription high fluoride toothpaste. He believed this would stave off the possible decay that the radiation and lack of saliva could cause.

The use of fluoride is one of those controversial topics, and I will not go into a great deal of detail about it. Most dentists will tell you that fluoride is safe and the benefits far out way the risks, especially during radiation treatment of the mouth and/or throat. However, there are dentists and other scientists who argue that the use of fluoride is dangerous and can cause cancer. You will have to decide for yourself where you stand on this.

My choice was to use the fluoride once a day and brush with the prescription toothpaste. I did this throughout my treatment and into my recovery and, so far, have no issues with my teeth.

During treatment, I began using a humidifier in my room at night and a mouth lubricating product called Biotene (there are many different products on the market for dry mouth). These things helped manage my dry mouth. Products for dry mouth come in liquids, sprays, and gum.

I also want to mention that sores in the mouth and on the tongue are common during radiation treatment. That being said, I was lucky to never have any. There are prescription and non-prescription products that can help with mouth and throat pain. For example, liquid lidocaine is often used for this and effectively numbs the mouth and throat.

If you are receiving radiation treatment directed at your mouth or throat, it is important to spend fifteen to twenty seconds each day inspecting your tongue and inside your mouth for abnormalities. This can save you major headaches later on. Seeing your dentist more often and immediately after treatment is concluded can also be a great preventative measure. If anything in your mouth looks out of the ordinary, see your doctor right away. Remember that for whatever reason during the cancer process, if a problem starts it seems to accelerate very quickly. That could be from the fact that treatment severely compromises our immune system so our bodies cannot put up much of a fight.

CHANGE OF IDENTITY

The treatment itself can feel dehumanizing. There are so many cancer patients and so many stories. The infusion room where I received my chemotherapy was always crowded. The oncologists, nurses, and technicians were always busy. Sometimes it seemed like everyone had cancer, and I was one of many people who would be seen and treated that day. Overall, I did have an excellent group of people working with me, from doctors to nurses to technicians. But there seemed to be so many of us cancer patients that it would be easy to forget the humanity part.

One of the challenging parts of treatment was feeling like my identity was slowly slipping away. What I looked like, felt like, and thought, all were changing. My face looked pale and gaunt. The only way I can describe it is looking skeleton-like. I had seen this look on others who had participated in chemotherapy. Eventually, the skin on my neck started to redden, dry, crack, and slough off. I was told it would feel and act like a sunburn, which it did. It wasn't painful, only itchy and annoying at times. The color in my face seemed off. I didn't recognize myself in the mirror. These were minor things compared to what could have happened, but it was disorienting just the same to not see myself anymore.

Dealing with the physical changes happening to me because of the treatment and with the sheer numbers of doctors, medical personnel, procedures, instructions, appointments, and so on, was understandably overwhelming. Sometimes I even felt as if it was someone else going through all of this. It was like I was in a dream, and none of it was really happening—that I had detached from "me" and had been replaced by someone else, this sick person whom I didn't recognize. I often had the fantasy that I would wake up having a second chance at life without having had cancer.

ALTERED SENSES

After the second week of radiation and chemotherapy, food started to taste terrible. I remember eating a slice of leftover pizza and thinking that somehow it must have spoiled.

I remember craving a hamburger, buying one, taking a single bite, and then throwing it away. That hamburger was the last food I would eat by mouth for the next five months. After treatment began, food tasted like cardboard that had been dragged through the mud and then doused with gasoline. Even water tasted this way.

All of my senses were altered as a result of treatment (I think due to the chemotherapy drug). This phenomenon was not something I was prepared for, understood, and, from what I gathered, may not have been that common. I would have occasional visual and auditory hallucinations. I saw glowing colors and floating cats at times. I heard someone talking or calling my name when there was no one around. Tactilely, I hated being touched, and it sometimes felt like an electrical current went through my body when someone touched me. I felt hot and cold at the same time and would turn an electric blanket on high, get under it, and still shiver. I even became confused as to whether I was actually hot or cold, so I couldn't figure out what I needed to do to remedy this.

My perception of time changed as I would often think that many hours had passed when it was only a few minutes. I got confused between night and day, dozing off and waking up thinking it was the middle of the night when it was the middle of the day. I was thankful my wife was there for me to keep me oriented enough so that I didn't miss appointments.

The smells were the worst. Everything and everyone smelled bad. If my wife cooked anything, I had to leave the room. As much as it pains me to say this, she smelled awful to me as well. This was hard for her. She wanted to comfort me, touch me, hug me, and be near me. I couldn't stand any of it.

During treatment, napping became a favorite activity. Being tired is a common side effect of both radiation and chemotherapy treatments. I was very tired and slept a lot. It wasn't until about three months after treatment that I slept less than ten hours a night. I have never in my life fallen asleep reading a book, and it was extremely rare for me to fall asleep watching TV. During treatment and soon after, I would and could sleep in any situation. I slept in doctors' waiting rooms, during chemotherapy, and while in the radiation tube receiving treatment. I even fell asleep mid-sentence in conversations with my wife. Luckily, she understood this and was not offended.

The radiation and the chemotherapy made me tired. I also was using a fentanyl patch, which was to control throat pain, and taking hydrocodone. These two drugs tired me out as well. If I were to be honest, I didn't need as much of these medications as were prescribed. I became used to the pain in my throat and only felt it when I swallowed, which was not very often. The truth is I used these medications more to help me relax and sleep and to escape.

Coincidentally, when I started using these medications during my treatment, it was at the height of the opioid crisis. I was afraid that somehow pain medication would be withheld from me, and I would suffer. Thankfully, this did not happen.

I also had the brief fear that I might become addicted to the medications. I decided that if I had to go through a drug rehabilitation program after treatment, I would be okay with that. It would be a small price to pay.

One of the most common side effects of hydrocodone (aka Norco) is constipation. This is commonly prescribed (at least when I was receiving treatment) to manage the throat pain resulting from the radiation treatments. Your doctors do not want you to become constipated. You will be questioned about this often, and you will be instructed to report it immediately if it becomes an issue.

Treatment often felt like a balancing act—how far can things be pushed, what will my body tolerate, and where is that line between killing the cancer and causing too much suffering to the patient. And your medical condition can change quickly, so giving accurate information and reporting concerns can be very important.

CHAPTER 7
MY FRIEND
THE FEEDING TUBE

HAVE MET THROAT cancer survivors who never had to use a feeding tube though I think this is rare. I have met others who had no issues with using their feeding tube and never had to use a pump (I will explain later what the pump does). I was not one of those people. I can't emphasize enough how much I hated my feeding tube. I also realize that it saved my life since I could not eat or drink anything by mouth for over five months.

There were many issues regarding my feeding tube, and I have to say that given all my experiences during my cancer process, dealing with my feeding tube and feeding formula were possibly the unanticipated worst. If I had known then what I know now, I would have done some things differently and thus had a less difficult experience. I seemed to have had more problems with the tube, the feeding process, and the feeding formula, than others who have had to live with a feeding tube.

There are a few different types of feeding tubes, and it is up to the doctors to decide the correct type for a patient. My tube was placed in my stomach about six inches above and an inch or so left (from my vantage point) of my navel. The tube stuck out about six inches and had a squeeze clamp on the end for opening and closing it. It was about a quarter inch in diameter. The tube had to be flushed with water daily when not in use and frequently (before and after feeding) when in use.

My tube was surgically placed, meaning I was put to sleep for insertion. The surgeon placed gauze and tape over the opening where the tube was inserted into my abdomen. The opening is called the stoma. When I woke up, the area where the tube was inserted was sore as expected. I was told it would be better in a few days. I noticed that my skin seemed to be reacting to the tape that held the gauze over the stoma. It was a large piece of tape called Tegaderm and used frequently in the medical field. They had shaved the area around the tube, and it quickly became red and itchy. No one had told me anything about stoma care or changing the gauze and tape. This was an oversight since I was supposed to have gone through some type of education program for feeding tube care and usage.

My skin became worse, and I had no idea how or if I could change the gauze and tape, so I went to urgent care. The doctor I saw was very nice but had no experience or knowledge about feeding tubes and stomas and was not sure what to do. She made some calls, and we waited for some answers. She was told she could remove the tape, clean the area around the stoma, and replace the tape. She was careful, and about four hours after coming in, I left knowing how to change the gauze and tape. I continued to have a skin reaction to the Tegaderm tape and changed to what is called paper tape, which caused less of a skin reaction. The tradeoff was that paper tape did not stick as well. Soon after this experience, I attended the feeding tube care and usage educational training I was supposed to have had sooner.

To use the tube, I could Bolus feed or use a pump. Bolus feeding is a method where I would fill a large plastic syringe with feeding formula (it held sixty milliliters maximum, or just over two ounces), insert the plastic needle part of the syringe into the feeding tube, and push the plunger, which would force the formula thorough my feeding tube and into my stomach. I can't really describe what that felt like. It was a bit of an odd sensation, especially if pushed in too quickly. When it became too painful to swallow and even liquids tasted terrible, I had to use the feeding tube to stay hydrated as well. I was told I needed somewhere around seventy ounces of water per day pushed into the tube.

I couldn't tolerate Bolus feeding very well. I would immediately feel dizzy, nauseous, and bloated. It hurt my stomach. My dietician suggested I inject the formula very slowly, maybe taking ten minutes to inject a single syringe full of formula or water.

I was instructed to consume eight boxes of the feeding formula per day. This was about sixty-four ounces total. In addition to this, I needed to have seventy ounces of water per day. All of this had to be taken through the feeding tube due to the issues I had with taste and increasing pain when swallowing. I had as much trouble tolerating the water through the feeding tube as I did the feeding formula.

If I was able to tolerate Bolus feeding by taking ten minutes for every two ounces of formula or water, it meant I needed to consume sixty-seven syringes of liquid per day. This amounted to a total of 670 minutes, or just over eleven hours per day of Bolus feeding. This was not possible.

64 ounces of formula per day
70 ounces of water per day
_____
Total liquid per day, 134 ounces

2 ounces for each Bolus feeding

134 ounces / 2 ounces per Bolus feeding = 67 Bolus tubes needed per day

67 Bolus's @ 10 minutes each = 670 minutes, or 11.1 hours of Bolus feeding.

I expressed this concern to the dietician and others but felt ignored. I kept being reminded how important hydration and calories were. Instead of pushing the issue, which is what I should have done, I resisted doing what I was told. By not speaking up, I ended up punishing myself. I didn't take in enough calories or water each day and quickly lost weight and became dehydrated.

There had been the option of using a feeding tube pump. A pump would attach to my feeding tube, and it would automatically direct formula into the tube very slowly, which I could tolerate. However, I was resistant to using it. It was not large or heavy, but inconvenient.

In order to consume enough feeding formula, I needed the feeding pump attached to my tube for roughly twenty hours per day, even while I was sleeping. If I tried to pump in the formula any faster than this, I felt sick. The pump seemed complicated to set up and temperamental to use and had to be carried around, and I didn't want that thing attached to me. My resistance to using the feeding pump also contributed to my losing weight and becoming dehydrated.

Soon after the second week of treatment, I went from being

able to eat by mouth to not being able to eat or drink anything. This happened quickly. I didn't have much of an appetite anyway, so I wasn't feeding myself much through my feeding tube because I didn't like it and didn't feel good after using it. I ended up in the emergency room due to stomach pain (issues with the feeding formula which I will discuss at length) and dehydration. After eight hours in the ER and several uncomfortable tests to make sure the tube was working and positioned correctly, I was hydrated and released. I was instructed to attend daily intravenous hydration sessions, which I attended six days per week for two to three hours per day for the next few months. Intravenous hydration should have been recommended from the beginning of my treatment. It seemed to help and is something I would suggest discussing with your doctor at the start of treatment.

I remember attending one of my weekly appointments with my radiation oncologist after I had lost weight quickly because I was not eating, drinking, or using my feeding tube very much. My radiation oncologist, my wife, and a nurse did an intervention. I understood the need for what they did, but it started with the radiation oncologist looking at my weight and then saying in a loud critical tone, "How about a little cooperation here?" He used the stick approach, reminding me of side effects, slowness of recovery if I didn't keep my weight on, and possible additional hospitalizations. I should have yelled back at him, "How about a little empathy here?"

I had many ongoing issues with the feeding tube, the feeding formula, and the site of insertion into my stomach. The insertion site was always painful and often red and tender. My skin did not like surgical tape of any kind and would easily become red and itchy. I didn't tolerate the formula well, so I had to use a feeding pump for twenty hours per day feeding very slowly as to not upset my stomach. When using the pump, I would often get the tubing caught on something, and it would pull and cause pain, further irritating the insertion site.

I had to sleep with the pump connected, which meant the tubing from the pump was connected to the tube that came out of my stomach. This connection between the two tubes was taped and often would leak or pull apart. The feeding formula was a sticky mess, and more than once I woke up in a puddle of it. I ruined some bed sheets, our sofa, and some of my clothes. There were always remnants of formula on the counter tops, sink handles, and floor. I even got some on my car seats and maybe my cats. I am pretty sure the formula would take the paint off of the walls, and this is what was keeping me alive.

When I left the house, I had to wear a backpack that was made to hold the pump and an IV bag full of formula. The tubing would exit the backpack, coming around my body, and disappear under the front of my shirt as it attached to the tube in my stomach. I carried this always. It was like having an annoying sibling who was always following me around creating problems. The pump made a low, distinct sound that became like a ringing in my ears that I could not get away from. Eventually, the sound faded into the background.

If the tube from the pump, which was about an eighth inch in diameter, became clogged somehow, the unit would shut off and start beeping loudly. And it became clogged a lot. The unit and the tubing were very temperamental. If something leaned on the pump, or it got propped up the wrong way, or if someone stepped on the tubing or it got caught on something, the pump would shut off and start beeping. If formula ran out, it would start beeping, and everything had to be reset.

Sometimes it seemed like the pump was in a bad mood and decided for no reason to shut itself off and start beeping. This meant I had to find the cause of the issue, and if I couldn't, I had to reset everything or start all over with a fresh set up.

Each day I had to have a new bag that would connect to the pump and new tubing in the backpack. It had to be threaded through a number of twists and turns. The pump had to be primed, and then it was attached to my feeding tube. It was about a fifteen- to twenty-minute process, but it felt like hours. Often something would not work correctly and have to be fixed or rethreaded, or I had to start completely over.

The IV bag connected to the pump would typically run out of formula about 5:00 a.m. each morning and beep until I woke up and turned it off. I would disconnect the pump and have a few hours' reprieve, which was a luxury. Then when I woke up again later, I would reconnect the pump and start using it again.

My wife started preparing the pump and backpack for me every morning. It was a small thing, her setting up my feeding backpack, but it seemed like such a huge relief. Small victories.

From the beginning of using the feeding formula, I had issues with tolerance. I was not even aware that how I was feeling had anything to do with the formula. I had attributed months of problems with the feeding formula as side effects of my chemotherapy and radiation. It was my naturopath who provided me with some information that changed everything. It is information the dieticians should have told me but never did.

The first discovery was that due to the amount of time I had to use the feeding pump, about twenty hours per day, my digestive system was never allowed to rest and recover. The very act of having to digest and process the formula, even while I was sleeping, kept my body and digestive system working hard around the clock. This effort my body had to make to digest the formula twenty hours per day was taxing enough, but imagine combining this with the effort it took for my body to recover from constant radiation and chemotherapy treatments. I was wearing myself out. Though I was sleeping, my body was not getting enough rest.

The second important discovery was that commercial feeding tube formulas are full of unhealthy ingredients, such as processed sugars and chemicals. No cancer doctor, cancer nurse, or dietician ever told me anything about overworking my body by feeding twenty hours a day or communicated any of the information I am about to share. It was not until I had been using the feeding tube and feeding formula for about five months that I learned what I am about to disclose. I am very thankful to my naturopath for helping me with this.

For a better understanding the issues that feeding formula can create, I need to provide some background information. When I was in treatment in 2017 and 2018, there were three categories of feeding formula available. All feeding tube formulas fit into one of these three categories. There were standard formulas, elemental formulas, and specialized formulas. Since many feeding tube patients must ingest all of their calories through their feeding tube, a formula is generally high in calories and has enough fat, proteins, and carbohydrates to meet nutritional needs. The first category of formulas, the standard formulas, are the most common, and in many cases, the only formula that is prescribed for a feeding tube patient. They are frequently the only category of formula that an insurance company will pay for. Standard formulas are inexpensive to make, easy to use, contain readily available ingredients, and have a long shelf life.

The following is a list of typical ingredients found in standard feeding tube formulas. This information was taken from the Oral Cancer Foundation's website at https://oralcancerfoundation.org.

CARBOHYDRATES:

- Corn syrup solids
- Maltodextrin
- Hydrolyzed cornstarch
- Glucose
- Fructose
- Sucrose
- Sugar alcohols

PROTEINS:

- Casein
- Whey protein concentrate
- Milk protein concentrate
- Soy protein isolate
- Lactalbumin
- Sodium, calcium, potassium, and magnesium caseinates

FATS:

- Soybean oil
- Corn oil
- Canola oil
- Palm kernel oil
- Medium chain triglycerides (MCT) oil
- Safflower oil
- High-oleic sunflower oil
- Borage oil
- Fish oil
- Monoglycerides
- Diglycerides
- Soy lecithin

There are many kinds of standard formulas, but generally they contain most or all of the ingredients listed. Each brand and type of formula also includes micronutrients, vitamins, and minerals.

The American Heart Association recommends that men do not eat more than thirty-six grams of sugar per day and women no more than twenty-five grams. In the feeding tube formula called Isosource 1.5, which is one of the formulas that was prescribed for me, there are forty-four grams of carbohydrates per 250 milliliter (8.45 ounce) box. These carbohydrates are not from starches or fiber but rather from simple sugar.

One Butterfinger candy bar also has forty-four grams of carbohydrates from simple sugars. I needed eight boxes of this formula per day, which meant forty-four grams of carbohydrates per box multiplied by eight boxes per day equals 352 grams of carbohydrates per day. This is equivalent to the sugar content of eight Butterfinger candy bars per day. Eight boxes of Isosource 1.5 contain 352 grams of sugar. Eight Butterfinger candy bars contain 352 grams of sugar. I do understand that the feeding formula also contained vitamins and nutrients as well whereas a Butterfinger candy bar does not, but I was surprised at the amount of sugar in the feeding formula.

Maltodextrin, another main ingredient in standard formulas, is a preservative, a thickener, and a filler, typically used in highly processed foods. It has no nutritious value, spikes blood sugar, and is generally made from genetically modified corn. It is inexpensive to produce and found in many commercially made foods.

There are also high amounts of protein in the feeding tube formulas. The Isosource 1.5 has seventeen grams of protein per 250 milliliters. Needing eight boxes per day, which incidentally is about 3000 calories per day, comes to 136 grams of protein per day. Is too much protein harmful to health? The consensus indicates it can be, and ironically too much protein has been linked to cancer.

How much is too much protein? There is a great deal of debate on the subject, and another book could be written about protein intake alone. Currently, the dietary reference intake guideline for protein intake recommends .36 grams of protein for each pound of body weight. For me, when I started treatment, this translated to a recommendation of 69 grams per day. I was consuming 136 grams per day. There is quite a range involved in the debate about what is a healthy amount. You will have to do your own research and decide for yourself.

It is also worth noting that the protein in the standard feeding tube formulas is from milk. Many people are allergic to milk products, which includes milk protein and whey protein, both of which are in standard feeding formulas.

There is a great deal of controversy and conflicting information about the healthiness of whey protein and dairy products in general. Health concerns center around the products themselves as well as how the products are processed. In general, dairy products are known to cause digestive and inflammatory issues for many people.

Soy products, also common in standard feeding tube formulas, are also controversial. Ironically, much of the information available links soy consumption to cancer (it is possible that this is because of how soy is typically grown and processed, rather than the soy itself).

So, the obvious irony to me is that these standard formulas are prescribed for the dietary needs of cancer patients and they contain high amounts of simple sugars (known to be unhealthy), high amounts of protein (believed to be linked to causing cancer), high amounts of dairy (known to cause allergic reactions in many individuals), and soy (also believed by some to be linked to cancer).

None of this was ever discussed by anyone, including any of the dieticians I spoke with, before or during my treatment. I only learned of this from the naturopath I saw after treatment, while I was still using my feeding tube.

The second class of feeding formulas are called elemental formulas. The short explanation of this type of formula is that they are supposed to be easier to digest due to having less fat in them and macronutrients that have been partially or fully broken down. If there is an absorption or digestive problem, this type of formula may be recommended. The typical ingredients in these formulas still contain maltodextrin, fructose, cornstarch, soy protein, casein (milk protein), and whey protein.

The third and last general category of feeding formula are specialized formulas. Individuals who have allergies to milk or whey or cannot tolerate the amount of sugar in the other types of formulas (due to diabetes, for example) may need specialized formulas. Specialized formulas can be produced that are organic, contain carbohydrates from vegetables (instead of from table sugar) and/or rice, are made with proteins from meat, beans, or vegetables instead of milk, and contain no soy products and little or no preservatives.

So, why aren't all formulas specialized? They could be made from all-natural ingredients and have enough calories and nutrients to meet the needs of feeding tube patients without using high amounts of sugars, milk proteins, or chemicals.

There are a few answers to this. All-natural formulas, ones that contain complex carbohydrates, can be slower and more difficult for the body to break down and digest. The body is extremely taxed by having to deal with cancer and treatment. The effort it takes to break down and use complex carbohydrates can overtax it. The standard and elemental formulas, though highly processed, may be easier for the body to use.

The other answer, the one I believe is the real reason the standard formulas are used, is cost. Specialized formulas are significantly more expensive to produce than standard formulas. The cost to consumers can be as much as six times the cost of the standard formulas.

The entire time I used standard feeding formulas I had problems. I tried many different standard formulas, and none of them were any easier for me to tolerate. I was told that the problems I was having (stomach pain, nausea, tiredness, bloating, etc.) were a result of chemotherapy and/or radiation. My naturopath was the only person who discussed with me the ingredients in the feeding formula and suggested it was the formula that was causing some of the issues I was having.

After five months of ingesting nothing but feeding formula, I had my cholesterol checked. My triglycerides, the level of fat in my blood, were 279. What is considered a healthy number for triglycerides is below 150. Before I started using a feeding tube, my triglycerides were 156. If all I had ingested for months was feeding formula, it had to be the formula that caused the elevation in my triglycerides. And it was from all the sugar I was ingesting.

I researched formulas and asked more questions. I read there are indeed people who have allergic reactions to feeding tube formulas called feeding tube intolerance. I had almost all of the listed symptoms. It is characterized by nausea, diarrhea or constipation, bloating, abdomen pain and/or discomfort, moodiness, and decreased energy. Similar to the possible side effects of chemotherapy and radiation except for the bloating and abdominal pain, my complaints were generally dismissed as the typical and usual side effects of my cancer treatment.

I spoke to a dietician and requested a specialized formula that was all natural. I was told that insurance would not cover this and that only in extreme cases, which were very rare, would an insurance company pay for specialized, or for that matter, elemental formulas. Standard formulas were what they paid for.

I spoke about this to a staff person at the local infusion center where I received my feeding formula and supplies. I was told that their contract for feeding formula in this area was with Nestle (yep, the chocolate company makes feeding formula), and they had to use Nestle products. At present they only produced standard formulas. I could try a different standard formula, but insurance would not cover any other type.

This is worth repeating. The feeding formula I was prescribed, Isosource 1.5, was made by Nestle and contained forty-four grams of simple sugars per box. Butterfinger candy bars are also made my Nestle and contain forty-four grams of simple sugars per bar. I was using eight boxes of Isosource per day.

I found some websites where all-natural feeding tube formulas were sold. They were made with real organic foods with no added sugars or maltodextrin and contained no milk proteins or soy. They were 100 percent natural and made with organic meats, beans, and/or rice and vegetables. They would meet both my nutritional needs and calorie needs.

These formulas were not cheap. I calculated that if I were to pay out of pocket, it would cost me about $1400.00 per month for the natural formula. This was about four times the out of pocket costs of the standard formulas, and the shelf life was less. My insurance would not pay for these formulas.

I purchased a sample box with my own money, just to try and see if I would feel differently. Sure enough, I tolerated this formula well. I made a comment about this to the infusion nurse where I received my feeding tube formula, and she informed me that if I stopped using the Nestle formula, they would have to take back my feeding pump and the backpack used for the pump. They would no longer be able to provide the supplies needed for the feeding tube and pump (feeding bags, tubing, stoma gauze, tape, bolus syringes, etc.). I would need to find and purchase all of these things on my own. I discovered that if I had to pay out of pocket for these things, my initial cost would be $1500 to $2000 for the pump and supplies in addition to $1400 per month for the natural formula and other ongoing monthly costs for supplies.

My naturopath suggested I make my own formula using a Vitamix blender. There were many websites that talked about making feeding formula using ingredients such as rice, lentils, garbanzo beans, and flax seed oil. I started listing combinations of ingredients in different volumes that matched the number of calories I needed to take in per box of formula as well as calculating the needed amounts of carbohydrates, fats, and protein. I could thin the mixture with water so that it would go through the bolus syringe and into my feeding tube. There were recipes online, and my naturopath helped me as well.

I first tried to make my own formula in a regular blender with no success. A regular blender would not break down the ingredients enough. I then purchased a Vitamix blender. The Vitamix was not cheap, about $350.00 for the most basic model, but it worked amazingly. It could liquify just about anything.

There were some trade-offs. Again, the standard formula was inexpensive (and because insurance covered this it cost me nothing) and easy to use, required no thinning, and had a long shelf life. However, it made me feel ill almost all of the time, and most of the ingredients were not healthy. The purchased natural formula was expensive and thicker. I had to thin it with water, reducing the caloric value, which meant I needed more of it to meet my calorie requirements. It also had less of a shelf life and would not last more than a few hours once opened (an opened container of standard formula was good for at least twenty-four hours).

The homemade formula was cheap to make and had healthy natural ingredients. However, the lentils, garbanzo beans, and rice had to be prepared first, measured out, and then mixed, which took more time and motivation and was messy. The mixture had a very limited shelf life and had to be thinned with water, so I needed more of it to meet my calorie needs. If it was stored in the refrigerator, it would become very thick, so I had to mix only what I was ready to use. I also couldn't use the homemade formula with my pump because I couldn't seem to get it quite thin enough. The tubing from the pump was slightly narrower than the feeding tube that came out of my stomach (this fact really didn't make any sense—the tubes should be the same diameter). But since I could tolerate the homemade formula well, I could use the bolus syringe to feed myself faster than the pump would.

I decided I would compromise. I would use some of the purchased natural formula, which I was able to tolerate so much better, some of the formula that I made myself, which I also tolerated well, and some of the standard formula that I was given.

As I changed what I was feeding myself, I was also able to change the amount of time per day I was feeding. I no longer had to attach the pump to myself while I slept. I was so tired of doing this (pun intended) that I didn't care if I had to deal with feeling sick by bolus feeding myself the standard formula on occasion. I was not going to use the pump while I slept anymore. I can't describe the feeling of freedom I had when I no longer had to sleep with the feeding pump running. It was a huge accomplishment.

Two important things happened. First, I felt better almost immediately. Not having the standard formula all of the time was a great step forward as was sleeping without my body having to work to all night digesting. Second, my throat was healing, and I could start drinking small amounts of liquid and eating ice chips for the first time in months. I started drinking apple and grape juice that I had frozen in ice trays. It was a good way to get some calories in and numb my throat. The more calories I could eat or drink, the less I had to use my feeding tube.

Things still didn't taste great, but there were a few things that were tolerable. I quickly moved on to making smoothies and eating soggy cereal. My daily meals began to be a combination of feeding formulas taken through the tube or bolus syringe and things I could eat or drink. Within a few weeks I was 100 percent eating again. Things tasted off, some things really bad, but I didn't really care since I felt better. All I wanted was that feeding tube out of me. After two weeks of eating by mouth and not needing my feeding tube, and after my PET scan showed that I was clear of cancer, the tube was removed.

SUGGESTIONS FOR DEALING WITH YOUR FEEDING TUBE

1. Pay close attention to your skin around the stoma and the stoma itself and its reaction to the tape that is used. Many people have reactions to the tape. There are different types available.

2. There is stoma powder available (I found it online) that can help ease some of the pain and itching or oozing that can occur.

3. There is also topical lidocaine available. I was prescribed this to ease the skin irritation that occurred on my neck due to the radiation. However, I often used it on my

stoma to ease the pain and itching, and it helped. Ask your doctor about it.

4. Keep your stoma clean. Since I had so much trouble with mine, it could become irritated easily. I changed the gauze (you will likely keep a piece of gauze over the stoma) at least twice a day and cleaned the stoma and area around it with a damp cloth with each gauze change.

5. Instead of using tape all of the time to keep the feeding tube from moving around under my shirt, I bought a feeding tube belt. It was called a TUUBEZZ Feeding Tube Belt that I found it online (https://www.tuubezz. com/). It fits like a belt around your waist under your shirt with Velcro and secures the feeding tube without having to use any tape. Remember my tube stuck out about six inches. There are tubes that are flush to the skin, and you won't need to secure these.

6. Start researching feeding formulas and consider supplementing the standard formulas with natural ones or with something you make yourself. Even if you tolerate the standard formulas, there remains the question regarding the healthiness of the ingredients. Recall that my triglycerides went way up as a result of the formula.

7. Be patient. I don't think that anything throughout my cancer, treatment, and recovery process tested my patience as much as having to deal with my feeding tube and pump. Not being patient doesn't help. Understand that you will spill formula and likely ruin some clothing, sheets, and maybe a sofa or chair.

8. Start seeing a naturopath. I wish I would have done

this sooner and started on some herbs/supplements that would have helped my stomach. Of course, share with your medical doctors what you are taking (to make sure the interactions between all of the drugs and supplements or herbs are safe) as well as your naturopath. I wish I would have started acupuncture as soon as I started treatment, (my naturopath also does acupuncture) which would have helped me relax more.

9. Keep a close eye on your supplies and how much formula you have. The feeding tube and supplies, which can include a pump and supplies for it, are literally your lifeline. Running out of needed formula or needed supplies (like bolus syringes or tubing for the pump, etc.) can mean you don't eat. Physical deterioration can happen very rapidly during treatment and having to miss a meal or meals can cause harm. I was lucky that the agency that supplied my formula and supplies was great. They constantly checked in with me when they thought I was ready for more formula or supplies. I was using eight boxes of feeding formula each day. That is fifty-six boxes per week or roughly 240 boxes per month.

10. If you use a feeding pump, keep it charged and take the cord with you when you leave the house. The pump, at least the one that I used, had a rechargeable battery. It would run for many hours without having to be plugged in. I sometimes would forget that it needed to be recharged, and the battery would die, and the pump would stop. This was problematic if I was not near a plug or didn't have the charging plug with me or if I was at an appointment.

11. If you use a pump, always carry tape and an extra pump bag/tubing unit and extra formula. The tube from the pump inserted into the feeding tube and was held together with tape. The tape would sometimes loosen or would need to be replaced. Sometimes the tube from the pump would clog and have to be replaced with a new bag/tubing unit.

12. If you wear the pump for a long period of time each day, give yourself a break from it. Again, small victories. The feeling of freedom I experienced when I had even a few hours without being tethered to the pump was pretty nice. It was a reward I would work toward and give myself. It sounds small and trivial when I write about it now, but it wasn't so when I experienced it. There is so much that doesn't feel good during the whole cancer process. It is so important to find the little things that make you feel good.

13. Entertain your food fantasies. After I was no longer able to eat, I started thinking about food constantly. I kept a food fantasy journal and read lots of recipe magazines. I had the strangest cravings for things I had not eaten for years: bologna sandwiches, canned Chef Boyardee ravioli, Kraft macaroni and cheese.... I kept a food journal of all of the things I wanted to eat when I could eat again. I had pages of things. I enjoyed reading recipe magazines (I called it my food porn) and collecting recipes I wanted to make when I could eat again. At some point, when I could deal with the smells of food again but still couldn't eat, I started to cook some meals for my wife. There I was in the kitchen wearing my feeding pump on my back or continually dragging it around the kitchen moving it

from counter to counter. Of course, I stepped on the tube occasionally by accident and then had to reset the pump.

One last discovery I made about my feeding tube and pump I want to share. There was a long-time during treatment when I did not want to be social. I didn't feel good. I slept a lot and had a very busy schedule with treatments, doctor's appointments, and self-care routines.

After I concluded radiation and chemotherapy, I still couldn't eat and still had a feeding tube. But eventually, I felt better and wanted to be social again. What I realized was that so much in our culture (and other cultures) centers around food. We socialize with others by having meals or going for drinks or coffee. Because I was still unable to eat, I had wrongly assumed I couldn't be social. If I went out for a meal or a drink or for coffee with others, I would have to sit there and watch, which made me and my companions uncomfortable.

In hindsight, I realize that I could have been more social anyway. I could have invited people over for a visit and offered them a snack or a drink. I could have gone out for short visits (it took a while for my stamina to come back) that didn't involve eating or drinking. This was an important thing for me to realize in that it allowed me to lean on my friends for support in my recovery and allowed me to feel more normal again. I did indeed attend some gatherings at restaurants or people's houses while I still had my feeding tube and could not eat or drink. It was a little awkward, and even though I said I was fine, I was a little resentful that I could not partake. However, I am glad I did it just to spend the time with people I cared about. When I was still using the pump, I would disconnect it for a few hours when I was with others if I could, just to feel more normal.

CHAPTER 8
RECOVERY

WHEN MY TREATMENT ENDED

R ADIATION AND CHEMOTHERAPY lasted six weeks. My last radiation treatment was November 30, 2017. I had completed chemotherapy a week before this. I started eating again without the aid of the feeding tube about four months after treatment ended toward the end of March 2018. The tube was removed in early April.

I considered my recovery to be everything that happened after my radiation and chemotherapy were completed. I also experienced two somewhat distinct phases of recovery.

Acute recovery was healing from the immediate consequences of radiation and chemotherapy. For me, acute recovery included: healing of the skin on my neck that was impacted by the radiation, lessening of the pain and discomfort in my throat, feeling less nauseous all of the time, being able to drink fluids by mouth, and eating again. For the sake of using some type of timeline, I would say that acute recovery began immediately after treatment and lasted several months.

Long-term recovery is likely to last a lifetime and includes healing from the psychological impact of the whole process and dealing with whatever long-term side effects that may or may not go away in the future. It also means dealing with anything that might happen in the future that is a result of the chemotherapy and/or radiation treatments.

I am not sure exactly where the acute phase ends and the long-term phase begins. I don't see the timing of this transition being terribly important other than being aware that some things will take longer to heal from than others, and some things may be changed forever. Like everything else about cancer and treatment, the recovery process will vary from individual to individual and is extremely difficult to predict. And like everything else involving cancer and treatment, it requires patience. It is likely that parts of recovery may take a lifetime. However, that does not necessarily mean that issues don't become easier and less intense. You are likely to experience a new normal, both physically and psychologically.

It is time to talk about one of the harder truths of treatment. This is something that will likely apply to everyone who goes through chemotherapy and/or radiation. The side effects of the radiation and chemotherapy treatments, at least right now in 2018 for throat cancer, are cumulative. By cumulative, I mean that the side effects seem to be at their worst when treatment ends. The typical protocol for throat cancer is around six weeks of treatment. Things were at their worst for me at almost exactly the six-week mark.

Throughout treatment I was told that if I ever started running a fever of more than 100 degrees that I needed to be seen by a doctor right away. This was never an issue until three days after my final radiation treatment (I had finished my chemotherapy treatments the prior week). I had already learned the hard way that one moment everything can be fine and then without warning a problem could progress rapidly. I developed a fever of over 100, so I went to the emergency room.

When you have cancer, you go to the front of the line. In

emergency rooms if you say you are in cancer treatment, you are seen right away—no waiting. If you call to speak with an oncology nurse and you are a patient, someone talks to you immediately. Cancer is the disease that allows you to be treated like royalty—kind of ironic.

I was seen almost immediately in the emergency room, and they ran some tests. I was told that my red and white cell counts were abnormal. They had been fine less than a week before, so this changed extremely fast. They wanted to admit me to the hospital so they could monitor me and get my cell counts under control. If I had this to do over again, I would have fought to stay out of the hospital. It was a terrible experience that didn't help me at all.

After spending some time in the emergency department, I was admitted to the hospital sometime after 1:00 a.m. At around 2:00 a.m. a nurse came in to check my vitals, set up an IV, and talk to me.

I mistakenly thought that hospitals were supposed to be places of comfort and care. In fact, one of the things that eased my mind about accepting treatment was knowing that if I needed to, I could go to the hospital. Both times I went to the emergency room during treatment, I left the hospital feeling worse than when I went in. I would now do everything I could to stay away from emergency rooms and hospitals.

I was not able to rest because at least every two hours I was awakened. The laboratory technician came to draw blood. The nurse came in to check my vitals or change my IV, or my IV medication would run out and the machine would beep loudly until someone came to reset the machine and/or change out my medications. It was not uncommon for the IV machine to beep for half an hour or more before someone came. And someone was in my room doing something at least every few hours, so sleeping was almost impossible.

I started having fits of coughing where I felt as if I was going to choke and had trouble breathing. I was being given medication every four hours, and without fail after three and a half hours, I started coughing again. I would call for a nurse, but often I had to wait a half hour or more for someone to come. A few times I thought I wouldn't stop choking.

I wanted out of the hospital and pleaded with the hospital physician to let me go home. After a few days, she released me. I should have set some boundaries with the staff and told them they needed to coordinate the times they checked on me, or I was not going to cooperate. I also should have said I would refuse to cooperate with blood draws or vital sign checks if I was not allowed to sleep for at least five hours.

Sleep deprivation made everything worse. I felt worse leaving the hospital than going in, but I was glad to be out. My instructions after being released from the hospital were to rest and recover, and daily for the next week or so, I had to return to the cancer infusion center for injections to help bring my white cell count back to normal.

It seemed odd to me that it was almost immediately after treatment ended that I was at one of the hardest points in the entire process. I was indeed experiencing all of the cumulative effects of the radiation and the chemotherapy. My throat was raw, and I was taking more pain medication than before. The good news was that the pain medications worked and made things tolerable. The bad news was that the pain medications wiped me out even more and made it hard to do anything but sleep.

The outside of my neck looked reptile-ish. It was burned like a bad sunburn—scaly, and peeling. It didn't hurt but was itchy and uncomfortable. I was told to use a moisturizing cream on it and also given a prescription for a topical lidocaine, which numbed my skin. My primary physician suggested A &

D ointment, which is typically used for diaper rash. It worked surprising well and cleared up my neck in a few days.

I still couldn't eat and had to manage my feeding tube and feeding pump. My body temperature was still off, and I couldn't tell if I was hot or cold most of the time. Strangely, I was often both at the same time. I would perspire and shiver simultaneously.

I remember asking my medical oncologist what I should do to help my body recover. She told me I needed rest. That was all the post treatment guidance I received from the traditional medical world, so I started doing more research on my own.

After my hospital stay, things started taking a turn for the better. The daily injections helped correct the issues with my white blood cell count, and I started feeling better. I was still anemic, which I was told would take time to improve.

My major goal at this point, aside from feeling better and not having cancer, was to have my feeding tube removed. My sense of taste had not returned, and swallowing was still difficult. My body was weak. I had lost thirty-five pounds and most of my muscle. I tired very easily.

I had my first big outing on New Year's Eve. My wife and I went to a friend's house. I ate a piece of shrimp, something I used to love, and it tasted terrible. I tried a sip of wine, which also tasted terrible. It would still be a while before I could eat or drink.

I had a good time but only lasted a few hours due to becoming tired. I met a man who had survived and recovered from stomach cancer. It was nice to hear a success story.

Sometime in January of 2018, which was about a month and a half after treatment ended, I started doing a few things that I am convinced helped my recovery tremendously. The first thing I did was to see a naturopath who had many ideas about how I could heal my body. I started taking supplements, probiotics, and other natural remedies that helped heal my immune system.

I also returned to my exercise class at the gym. This was hard. The overall temperature in the gym was kept on the cool side. I would sit and shiver though I was wearing layers of clothing and a down jacket. I was still dealing with being anemic, having low energy, and not having much muscle mass left. I remember the first several times I went. The extent of my routine was sitting in a chair and lifting each leg up and down for fifteen repetitions. After doing this for a few sets, I was exhausted, so I sat and watched everyone else for the rest of the time, or I would go sit in the car with the heater on.

Soon, I was able to add in more exercises (I went twice a week), and I could see I was progressing. I still had my feeding tube in and had to be very careful about lifting or doing anything that would strain my abdominal muscles. Slowly, I was gaining strength back. My trainer told me it would probably take about a year to gain back the muscle I had lost, and that was about how long it took. However, each time I went to the gym, I was able to do a little more.

The other thing I started doing sometime in January was seeing a mental health therapist. I was frustrated, angry, and scared. I had not yet found out if my cancer was gone. I still had my feeding tube and feeding pump and was discovering that my feeling bad physically was mostly due to my reaction to the feeding formula. I still had no idea how long I would have to use the tube. Food still tasted terrible, and my mouth was always dry. I realized going to Mexico in March for a vacation, as my wife and I had wanted to do, was probably not going to happen.

In late January, I returned to work. About six of the clients whom I had been seeing when I shut down my practice at the end of September, returned. I saw two clients a day—Tuesdays, Wednesdays, and Thursdays.

This was another lesson for me about patience. I returned to work too early. I had underestimated my stamina. I didn't have as much as I thought I did. Seeing two clients in a day was absolutely exhausting. I still needed ten to twelve hours per night of sleep and was still tired during the day.

I want to give some advice here. Listen to your body during treatment and particularly during recovery. Pushing through fatigue will only slow your recovery. Treatment is a total assault on your body, and your body needs time to heal. This sounds obvious, but it is something I would forget at times. If I needed rest, I would rest. If I needed ten to twelve hours of sleep each night, that is what I needed. Over time I have needed less sleep, but I still need more than I did prior to cancer.

I had a hard time remembering that the end of treatment was only the beginning of recovery, and that recovery can take a long time and depends on many factors. I also had to remember that recovery is not necessarily a linear process. Sometimes there are setbacks. I found it important to listen to what my body was telling me.

Cancer and treatment compromise our stamina and tolerance for psychological and emotional issues as well. It can be more difficult to deal with stress and emotions during treatment and recovery. Treatment weakens our bodies and our minds.

I found that during treatment and recovery I could easily become more impatient than usual, quick to anger, more judgmental, and more emotional. For a long time, I could not even hear the word cancer without having a physical and psychological reaction. I found myself listening to my clients' problems, and rather than feeling compassionate, I would feel judgmental, thinking things like "Really? That is your problem? I had cancer, and you complain about X?"

Rather than beating myself up about these things, I realized these were all signs of a worn psyche. Just as being tired was about a worn-out body, my mind was healing as well. Just as I had to listen to my body, I had to listen to my mind and take care of it. Seeing a therapist was one way I did this. Not putting myself into stressful situations was another. Limiting the number of clients I would see and how many hours I would work, was yet another.

Again, trying to push through the physical or the emotional healing that must occur only serves to delay the process. A "just get over it" attitude will only hinder recovery.

PET SCAN (NUMBER 2)

You may recall that a PET scan is a full body imaging process that, among other things, can detect cells in the body that may be cancerous. The doctors wanted to make sure there was no cancer remaining in my body. I had to wait about three months after treatment ended to have another PET scan. It takes about three months to be sure that the inflammation caused by the radiation treatments does not show up as a false positive during the PET scan.

This process was the same as my initial scan, but I was just as scared—not so much about the test itself, but of the results. I wanted to be cancer free.

The evening after my PET scan, my radiation oncologist left me a phone message. Being careful to never use words such as cured or cancer free, he said the scan looked good, significantly better than my first. There was still some activity showing in my throat, but he was sure this was a result of scar tissue caused by the radiation. He congratulated me. This was as close to saying I was cured as he could get.

PORT REMOVAL

After the PET scan showed there was no cancer in my body, it was time to remove the port. Removal of the port was like the insertion. I was taken into an operating room, and a drape was put over my chest and face. A surgeon numbed the area around the port by injecting lidocaine. He made an incision and removed it. I was awake and alert during the process but did not feel anything. He talked about playing golf to his assistant while he cut open my chest. He used glue to seal the incision, and the glue wore off in a few weeks. There was some itching around the incision as the glue dried and flaked off. It did leave a small scar just as the incision for the port placement did.

FEEDING TUBE REMOVAL

One of the best days of my recovery was the day I finally had my feeding tube removed, and I had no idea how this would be done. The doctor who had put in it was no longer inserting or removing them, so I had to find another physician who would remove it. How a tube is removed depends on the type that was inserted. Evidently, the only way mine was coming out was to pull it hard and fast. My tube was held in place with a rubber cap which was molded around the tube itself so the tube would not slide around. This cap rested against the inside of my stomach wall. The cap was not very big in diameter, but it was significantly larger than the quarter inch hole in my abdomen that the tube passed through. If the tube was pulled hard, the cap would fold like a mushroom and then forcibly pass through the opening. I had accidentally caught my feeding tube on many things during the time I had it and consequently had pulled on it pretty hard. This caused pain and discomfort, but it never felt like it would come out. It was difficult to imagine the tube being pulled out of me. I had no idea if I would be sedated for this, if the area around the tube would be numbed, or how the doctor would get that thing out.

I was nervous. Thankfully, the nurse navigator, whom I had met when I first had my feeding tube inserted, was there with me as I was about to have it removed. We chatted for what seemed like forever as I waited for the doctor to perform one of my last rites of passage into recovery.

The doctor examined my feeding tube and the stoma around it and said that numbing the area, which would require injections, would hurt much more than pulling it out. He wrapped the tube around his hands, told me to take a breath, and pulled hard and fast. I heard it literally snap out like a big rubber band. It felt like a bee sting. A quick, sharp pain that for some reason caused me to laugh and double over at the same time, and then I was fine. There was very little bleeding, and within a few hours, the hole in my stomach started to close up on its own and began to heal. I was so thrilled to have that six-month-old extra appendage out of me. This too left a scar, kind of like a second belly button. Another reminder of my cancer.

CHAPTER 9
SIDE EFFECTS
AND ANNOYANCES
AFTER TREATMENT

THE RETURN OF TASTE AND SALIVA

HAD ASSUMED THAT soon after treatment my taste buds would be back to normal. This was not the case. It has been a slow and unpredictable process that continues to evolve and change. It can't be accurately determined when you will be able to swallow again (if that was an issue), when the throat pain will go away, or when your feeding tube will come out (if you had one). I was told that three to six months after treatment is typically when you can eat again by mouth, food doesn't taste terrible, and the pain in your throat is gone. This will vary. For me, it was almost exactly four months after treatment that I was able to eat again, experienced no throat pain, and had my feeding tube removed. I have known others who have healed much faster and still others who have healed much slower.

Taste will probably take longer to return, and it can be a slow process. There will likely be a new normal here. I did not enjoy the taste of many things even though I could eat again, and then each month I noticed some things would taste a little better. Taste buds returning is an unpredictable process that can happen quickly, occur over a period of years, or not improve at all. For me, I would say that my taste buds were probably ninety percent back after a year. However, there are a number of foods I used to love that don't taste good anymore. I used to love any type of fruit, and now for some reason there is no fruit that tastes good to me. I was neutral about other foods before treatment that I enjoy more now. I have never been much of a beer drinker, but I have found that post treatment beer tastes better to me. I am very thankful that I can taste what I can.

Dry mouth is a common issue during and after treatment. Radiation damages saliva glands. How much damage, short- and long-term, will vary. Typically, like taste, saliva production will recover over time. There can be some difficulty with this process. For many, when saliva production begins again, it still may be difficult to swallow. The saliva is often thick and stringy and honestly hard to deal with (and can be a little disgusting). It is not uncommon for someone to have to spit into a cup or garbage container for a period of time while things heal. Just like everything else in this process, the severity of this and the time needed for recovery will vary.

I had only a short time, maybe a few days to a week, of dealing with thick saliva and was always able to swallow. Thankfully these were not major issues. For some people the above issues can take months or years to improve. For others it can happen much faster. I know survivors who must always carry water with them and constantly drink in order to keep their mouth moist. For me, I am still noticing small improvements. When I first could eat, I always had to have water in order to swallow. Now I only have to have water if I am eating bread or crackers, but I can eat pretty much anything else without having liquid with it. My mouth is still much drier than it was before treatment, and I still use a humidifier at night. If someone held a gun to my head and told me to spit, I couldn't do it. However, it is tolerable, part of my new normal, and the good news is that if it doesn't improve, I will never have to worry about drooling as I age.

During treatment I had lost thirty-five pounds, and all my clothes were too big. I was hesitant to buy many new ones since I had no idea where my weight would settle. I had always had a heavy five o'clock shadow. I had to shave my face and neck daily, or my beard would grow quickly. I also had a fair amount of hair on my chest. The radiation took care of all of that for me. My face and neck became extremely smooth. My chest was bare down to just blow my clavicle. My hairline on the back of my neck was about an inch higher than it used to be. These were all the areas that the radiation targeted.

After six months or so into recovery, the hair on my face started to grow again, and I had to shave. The hair on my neck and chest has not grown back at all. I am guessing it will not.

About a month or so into my recovery, I no longer needed the pain medications, so I stopped using them. I had been told I would need to taper off, but I didn't listen and did it my way. Not the best idea. I did have some withdrawal symptoms, but I didn't care. It was tolerable, and I felt like I wanted to be done with them.

THRUSH

One of the many possible side effects of cancer treatment, particular radiation to the mouth, is oral thrush. This was something I didn't pay much attention to until I had it bad. Oral thrush is an overgrowth of yeast or Candida, which we all have naturally in our bodies, that occurs on the tongue and/or in the throat. I found it to be disgusting and uncomfortable. It literally looked like a fur coat had grown on my tongue. It further increased my dislike for the taste of food and was an awful experience.

I won't go into the gory details, but if you are interested, there are many places online where you can look up symptoms or even see photos. It is a common occurrence with head and neck cancer patients and others whose immune systems are compromised.

Toward the beginning of treatment, I was told about the possibility of thrush. One of the many things I was told to do during treatment was to check my tongue and mouth daily. It was something I stopped doing, and it would have taken me about fifteen seconds a day. Before my medical oncologist saw I had thrush, I had assumed that what I felt in my mouth was a side effect of chemotherapy or radiation. Well, the thrush technically was, but if I had been more diligent and caught it earlier, I might have not gotten such a bad case.

My medical oncologist assured me it was common and not dangerous, just annoying. She prescribed me a week's worth of medication. The medication, which is commonly used for thrush, was called Fluconazole. It was not an easy medication for me because I had some side effects from it, but I figured it was only for a week. However, the thrush did not go away. In fact, it lasted through treatment and into recovery, almost six months total. It lived through my treatment of Fluconazole, a four times per day regiment of lozenges, two rounds of a four times per day liquid rinse called Nystatin, and then a two-week double dose of Fluconazole. After all of that, the thrush was still there.

It was highly contagious as well. When I was eating again, I could never use a utensil that my wife used and couldn't taste any of her food for fear of spreading the thrush. We could not drink out of the same glass or bottle and, of course, could not kiss.

Ten months post treatment, there were still traces of thrush, but it was almost totally gone from my tongue. Blood testing showed that I still have a lot of Candida in my system. I have tried a variety of herbal supplements that are supposed to help with this, but only more time will help it lessen.

LYMPHEDEMA

Lymphedema in the neck is swelling of the neck due to damaged lymph nodes and is a common side effect of radiation treatment. The lymphatic system is a network of vessels that run through the body. These vessels route fluids through the lymph nodes, which act as a filter for fluids and waste. There are over 500 lymph nodes in the human body.

It is common for radiation, and sometimes the cancer itself, to damage one or more lymph nodes. The American Head and Neck Society estimates that as many as seventy-five percent of those who receive radiation for head and neck cancer will develop some type of lymphedema.

When a lymph node is damaged, fluid cannot run through it, so the fluid becomes backed up. This can manifest as swelling, stiffness, and pain. If the damaged lymph node(s) is in your neck, it can cause changes in your voice, difficulty swallowing and, in severe cases, difficulty breathing.

Lymphedema is treatable and manageable. When my medical oncologist noticed I had it (my neck remained swollen after treatment), she referred me to a physical therapist who specialized in lymphedema treatment. The physical therapist showed me a number of massage techniques I could perform on my neck, which would manually move the fluid that was stuck. I was to do these daily (you can find videos on how to do this on YouTube).

She also recommended a neck compression garment. If

you search on the internet for "head and neck compression garments for lymphedema", you will find these for purchase. The most common one looks like a hijab, the head cover and scarf that Islamic women wear. However, the compression garment is made out of what feels like a panty hose material and is flesh-colored, and it compresses the neck, feeling to me like it constricts my airway. Not only is it odd looking, I found it very uncomfortable. I was supposed to wear this a few hours each day and sleep in it at night. I tried it a few times and gave up.

I asked my physical therapist to point me to studies that showed the use of the compression garment for lymphedema of the neck was an effective treatment. She said there are a number of studies that show compression helps with lymphedema located elsewhere in the body, but she knew of no studies that specifically addressed the effectiveness of neck compression in treating head and neck lymphedema. Yet using a compression garment was a standard treatment, along with massage, neck exercises, and skin care, for lymphedema of the neck.

My sessions with the physical therapist were weekly and lasted an hour. The first fifteen to twenty minutes she spent at her computer asking me the required insurance questions. On a scale of one to ten how much does your lymphedema cause you daily pain? How much would you say your lymphedema impacts your range of motion? How does your lymphedema...? I politely asked her if we could forgo the question/answer session or if she would at least make eye contact with me as she talked rather than looking at her computer screen. She explained that she was required to see at least six patients per day and what she asked me was required information for each patient. She was also expected to make notes on each one-hour session. The only way she could possibly complete these tasks was to do some of her computer work with each patient at the beginning of each appointment.

The remaining time of our appointment was spent with her teaching me and reviewing massage techniques for my face and neck. After about the fourth appointment, I had learned the massage techniques. After trying the compression garment a number of times, I made the decision I was not going to use it. It looked ridiculous and was uncomfortable, and there was no way I could sleep in it. If the lymphedema worsened, I would revisit my choice.

When I received my first explanation of benefits which listed the charges for the physical therapist, I was a little shocked. Each one-hour appointment was billed at around $600.00. My out of pocket portion was about $75.00 per session. It was not worth it to me since I now knew how to do my own neck massage, so I stopped going.

I discovered a local massage therapist who was a cancer survivor, and she specialized in massage for lymphedema. She charged $65.00 per hour and spent the entire hour working on my neck.

I saw her four or five times and felt like my lymphedema was under control. It could never be cured, only managed. I experienced a mild form with the only symptom being minor swelling of my neck (no pain, no difficulty swallowing, no range of motion issues, no stiffness), and it would come and go, often without reason. I decided I didn't want to commit the time and money long term for something that was not that bothersome, and I could work on myself. I figured if ever it got worse, I could seek her help at that time. I am not saying this decision is the right one or the one that might be right for you. It is simply the decision that I made for myself.

THYROID

About six months or so after my treatment ended, I noticed that I felt really good and had a great deal of energy. I needed less sleep, could concentrate well, and could work on and finish a number of different projects. When people asked me how I was doing, I joked that the radiation treatments must had supercharged me and may had given me superpowers.

This lasted for a month or two, and then slowly I lost this energy. In fact, I started feeling tired, needed more sleep, and had trouble concentrating. My weight, which had stayed stable after treatment, started creeping up for no real reason. I was cold all of the time, and my joints were sore.

You may have already figured out that after my energy dropped, I was exhibiting the classic signs of hypothyroidism, a thyroid that was not working. In August 2018, nine months after my treatment ended, I had my blood drawn specifically to check my thyroid function.

Understanding the results of the thyroid testing seemed complicated. A number of tests measure how it is functioning—TPO, T4, T3, and TSH to name a few. I do not totally understand how they all work together, and this is not the place to explain it all. I will say that all of these are indicators of how the thyroid functions and have to do with processes that involve the thyroid. My TSH, which was supposed to be between .4 and 4.0, was 24.3. My TPO, which was supposed to be between 0 and 34, was 490. I didn't have to understand much about these tests to see that something was way off. When I looked up abnormally high TSH and TPO, the indication was that I had severe hypothyroidism.

My thyroid had stopped functioning. The radiation had destroyed it. Before or during treatment, I don't recall anyone telling me this could be an issue. In researching this issue, seventy-five percent of throat cancer patients who were treated with radiation experience hypothyroidism. When I mentioned this issue in my head and neck cancer support group, everyone there seemed to have thyroid problems as a result of their treatment. Why is this not monitored? This should be a standard part of follow-up care after radiation treatment of the neck.

After I received the results of my thyroid testing, I made an appointment to see an endocrinologist, a doctor who specializes in dealing with thyroid issues and other parts of the body's endocrine system. After she reviewed my test results, she could see that my thyroid was not functioning. I began taking thyroid medication, which has helped tremendously. I take a small pill each morning and will do so for the rest of my life. I am still in the process of tweaking the right dosage, which involves a bit of trial and error. I take the medication for about four weeks and then have my blood tested. Based on the results of the testing, the dosage may be increased or decreased. I continue taking the medication for another four weeks and test again. I also monitor how I feel. Are the symptoms going away, staying the same, or changing?

She also told me something that surprised me. She had looked up the blood test that was done soon after my treatment had ended. My primary physician had done blood work and included a thyroid test. Based on her review of these results, she said I had an overactive thyroid at that time. That was the time when I felt I had unlimited energy and had joked I had been supercharged. This was something my primary physician missed.

My endocrinologist explained to me why I went from hyperthyroid (thyroid overworking, which gave me lots of energy) to hypothyroid (my thyroid not working, which left me with very little energy) within a few months. I don't remember the details, but given my treatment and its effect on my body, it made sense and was not that uncommon. It was like my thyroid knew it was dying and made some last-ditch effort to save itself by over-producing hormones. I miss the hyperthyroid days. It felt great to have the energy and clarity I felt.

So, my advice is simple. Soon after radiation treatment is complete, have your thyroid checked. Then have it checked regularly after that. The frequency will depend on what is happening, but don't assume that symptoms of anxiety, agitation, increased energy, and sudden weight loss (all symptoms of hyperthyroidism) or decreased energy, muscle aches, unexplained weight gain, and being cold most of the time (all symptoms of hypothyroidism) are simply normal side effects from the treatment. Thyroid damage can occur soon after treatment or years after treatment. This is why it is good practice to have it checked regularly.

TEETH AND MOUTH

There are things in life you will likely never think about unless you have to. I never thought about my taste buds and never gave any thought to saliva production. These are things treatment will impact. Issues may be short-term, or they may be long-term. Any radiation around the mouth/neck area will likely affect saliva glands and taste buds.

Soon after treatment, I returned to my dentist for a checkup, and my teeth were in good shape. I had mixed feelings about continuing to use so much fluoride, so I stopped the daily fluoride treatments but continued to use the high fluoride toothpaste. I see the dentist more frequently to make sure my teeth and gums remain healthy.

About a month or so into recovery, I felt something between two of my teeth. I could not get it out using regular dental floss, so I purchased a metal dental pick like my dentist uses. What I managed to remove was a piece of one of my teeth. I was discouraged and scared. I feared the radiation had damaged my teeth to the point that they would crack and fall out. I saved the piece of tooth and went to my dentist. It turned out it was a tooth colored filling that had broken off. It was a large filling and could easily have been mistaken for a piece of tooth. The filling had nothing to do with my cancer treatment and was easily replaced.

I would say that about eighty to ninety percent of my saliva production has returned. This is good news for my teeth. I definitely take better care of them now and make sure I don't miss any dental appointments.

Though my taste buds have mostly returned, many foods taste different than they used to. Things that I used to like— pizza, spaghetti, chicken, and fruit—all taste different. They don't taste right to me. However, other things do taste okay, and some even taste good. I see the alteration of my taste buds, which may or may not be permanent, as a small price to pay for still being alive. I also am aware that they continue to improve.

I do have some scar tissue in my throat as a result of the radiation. Massaging my neck helps break up the tissue. This is also minor, and most of the time I don't even notice it. I feel it only when I think about it and swallow. The hardest part about this is remembering that it is ONLY scar tissue and NOT tumors that have grown back.

HEAVY METAL TOXICITY

I had a heavy metals test done about six months after treatment. The result of the test indicated I have a fair amount of platinum in my system. This is a direct result of the chemotherapy drug, Cisplatin.

This was something that I recall no traditional Western-trained doctor mentioned, the potential of platinum staying in my system. My naturopath recommended that I be tested for heavy metals.

Heavy metals in the body are never good. They can cause cancer and a host of other neurological issues. This brings me to another irony of cancer treatment. The treatments for cancer, radiation and chemotherapy drugs, the very things that cure the cancer, can also cause cancer.

The long-term consequences of heavy metal toxicity build-up and of the radiation are not the same for each person. Just like everything else with cancer and treatment, the impact and how the impact may be managed will vary. I am still researching the potential impact of my treatment and what things I might do to correct or prevent future damage. I am working with my naturopath on using supplements to help flush out the platinum in my system.

Even though the effects of my treatment may cause problems in the future, the impact of not having the treatment was clear to me. I would not be here writing this now had I not had treatment. That I am sure about.

CHAPTER 10
RECOMMENDATIONS DURING RECOVERY

Surprisingly, when treatment ended, there was very little information and support from my treatment team as to how to build myself back up. To heal, I was told to rest, and they would follow up with me to make sure the cancer was gone. That was about it. I would imagine this will vary depending upon where you receive treatment and your medical team. I believe that how you care for yourself during recovery is as important as how you cared for yourself during treatment.

Based on my experiences, I would make the following recommendations. These may be things your medical team doesn't talk about, so it might be up to you to start conversations or find a physician who will help you with these recommendations.

THYROID CHECK

I would recommend getting your thyroid checked a few months after treatment ends and at least every six months after that. For me within about a six-month period following treatment, my thyroid stimulating hormone level (TSH) went from 0.6 to 24.3. TSH is a measure used to gauge thyroid function. I was told my ideal range should be between 1.0 and 3.0.

As I discussed earlier, it is very common for radiation treatment to impair the functioning of the thyroid. This could happen right away after treatment or sometime in the future, so a routine check of your thyroid is helpful.

I found it is also important to make sure your physician understands and pays attention to your thyroid test results. This may mean finding a specialist. My early blood work showed without a doubt that my thyroid was not functioning properly. My primary physician told me it was nothing to worry about and ignored it. When I saw an endocrinologist months later, she reviewed my past blood test results and could see that problems were beginning. Knowing this could have saved me some months of discomfort.

COMPLETE BLOOD PANELS

I think it is important to have complete blood panel done soon after treatment, and then at regular intervals. Treatment can throw many things off in your body. Remember, chemotherapy is putting poison into your system and killing cells. It will take time for your body to recover.

You will likely want to have a complete blood panel done with some regularity. Chances are pretty good that when you first have it done after treatment has ended, there will be some issues. As I have already discussed, I had issues with my red and white cell counts, my thyroid hormone, my triglycerides, and some other numbers that were off. This is where I worked with my naturopath and physician to take whatever medication and/ or supplements were recommended in order to correct these issues. The typical regime has been to have my blood tested, try whatever medications or supplements for four to six weeks, and then test again. I am still participating in this process.

Again, make sure that whoever is reading your blood work gives you an accurate interpretation and doesn't say everything is fine when it is not. It is important to do your own research as to what your numbers mean and ask your doctor about them.

HEAVY METAL CHECKS

It is advisable to have your blood tested for heavy metals three to six months after treatment and to consider a heavy metals detoxification process if needed. This is typically not a western medicine thing but generally ordered by a naturopath or herbalist. As I discussed earlier, no western physician said anything to me about heavy metal build up, yet it was there and can be dangerous.

Treatments for heavy metal toxicity range from taking special medications that bind with heavy metals (called chelators) to using herbs and minerals to detoxify the liver. Left untreated, heavy metal build up in your system can lead to all sorts of future issues, including cancer. It seems at least worth a conversation with a professional regarding potential risks and treatment.

PROBIOTICS / IMMUNE SYSTEM BOOSTERS

My naturopath recommended that I take probiotics and other supplements to repair internal inflammation and help strengthen my immune system. I am convinced that using probiotics during recovery was extremely helpful for getting my stomach back on track. There were so many drugs that went into my system during treatment that it made sense to me that the functioning of my stomach and digestive system were impacted. Taking probiotics helped my stomach return to normal and also helped with the nausea and indigestion I was experiencing. This is something to talk to your physician or naturopath about.

SLEEP

You will likely need a great deal of sleep. As I discussed before, it is important to listen to your body and not try to push through fatigue during recovery. Needing more sleep than you did prior to treatment is common. Sometimes this is a long-term thing, and sometimes it will only be for a short time. However, I believe that not getting enough rest and sleep can slow down and impede recovery.

It took six months to a year for my stamina to return. I went back to work two months after treatment was finished, and in hindsight that was too soon for me. I was exhausted most of the time and had to cut back my hours.

The key is to pay attention to your body. If it needs to rest, respect that and don't fight it. It has nothing to do with your character or your toughness. It is simply the fact that your body (and mind) have been traumatized by cancer and treatment. And like cancer and treatment, your need for rest and sleep may be different from others.

DENTAL

I've discussed the importance of caring for your teeth and mouth. This is something that will likely be long-term. Before treatment, I used to see the dentist every six months. Sometimes I would forget and go a year or more between visits. This never presented much of an issue for me but not so anymore.

Due to the radiation and possible long-term damage to my salivary glands, my teeth will be much more susceptible to decay. I saw the dentist right after treatment, and then every three months for the first year after treatment. Things are looking okay, so I am now seeing him every six months and I will make sure I keep these appointments.

Unfortunately, problems with your teeth, gums, jaw, and

mouth, can show up right away, or months or years down the road. It is important to keep on top of this by having regular checkups.

PRIMARY SITE CHECKS EVERY THREE MONTHS

Every three months for the first two years after treatment, and then every six months for three years after that, I will see my ENT who will use a scope to look into my throat. This is where he first saw the tumors before treatment, and where he saw they were gone after treatment. So far everything looks good. The tumors are gone and have not returned. If something were to return (though the recurrence rate is extremely low), catching it early is the best chance of intervention.

DETOX YOUR LIFE

After having cancer, I have become much more conscious about all the things I come in contact with on a daily basis that contain cancer causing agents, or at the very least contain questionable ingredients. This includes deodorants, shampoos, toothpaste, laundry detergents, household cleaning products, the coating on cooking pans, soaps, skin products, plastic containers, and food. All of these products contain or can contain dangerous chemicals, many of which have been proven to be carcinogenic.

During my recovery, I made some changes in these areas. I now use only natural/non-toxic deodorants, shampoo, toothpaste, face cream, laundry detergent, and household cleaning products. We got rid of our plastic food storage containers and purchased glass instead.

I am much more careful about what I eat and try to stay away from highly processed foods. I always read the ingredients on food labels and try to buy organic. Any store or co-op that sells natural products should carry these non-toxic alternatives. There are also many places online where you can purchase them as well.

I have no idea what difference this all will make, but I know that it can't hurt. There are many products that do contain toxic chemicals and avoiding them can only help. I also feel better knowing I am taking steps to stay healthier.

I also examined my relationships for toxicity. I asked myself if I found each relationship stressful and why. As I worked to detox the chemicals in my environment, I worked to detox the relationships in my life. In some instances, this meant walking away from friendships.

Cancer taught me how quickly life can change and how there may not be a tomorrow. Realizing that, why would I want to be around people whom I don't enjoy? Think of it this way, if you found out you had twenty-four hours to live, what would you do with your time? Would you be around people who you find stressful? Would you argue, complain, or try to change others?

I made clearer decisions about what I wanted to do with my time and who I wanted to spend it with. If I found there were those in my life whom I found stressful to be around, I would either not be around them anymore, reduce how much time I was around them, or simply work on emotionally letting go (if I couldn't avoid the person). I wasn't rude about it with anyone, just clearer about what I would and would not do.

Psychologically, it is very important to have positive, caring people in your life. As I said earlier, dealing with cancer will allow you to form bonds with people that you never thought would happen. Some people I barely knew or didn't know stepped up and were there for me. Others whom I knew, and even friends I had for a long time, simply disappeared. And others, who were trying to be helpful, but were not, I walked away from.

DIET AND EXERCISE

I believe that diet and exercise are extremely important, and even more so once you have had cancer. Admittedly, this is hard, but I have worked to clean up my diet and make sure that I exercise. Since I have had cancer once, I feel more susceptible which makes it more important than ever to be as healthy as I can.

SUPPORT

As I have discussed, the cancer process impacts our psyche. Many people assume that once treatment ends, the psychological impact of the cancer process is no longer an issue. This is not necessarily the case. Psychological issues can continue or resurface months or even years after treatment has ended. Simply knowing this can be helpful. Therapy, grief groups, and support groups, can be as important months or years after treatment as they are during treatment. In my local head and neck cancer support group there are people who are starting treatment, people who have recently completed treatment, and people who finished treatment years ago. The benefits of support do not expire.

CHAPTER 11
THE FINANCIAL IMPACT

I T IS SAD to me that there are still people who can't afford cancer treatment or those who must incur significant debt in order to be treated. The costs are staggering.

As an example, in October and November of 2017, I had thirty-three radiation treatments to my throat and neck. The billed amount for each treatment was $3000 which amounts to $99,000 total for my radiation treatments. My initial half hour consultation with my medical oncologist was $550. My twenty-minute post treatment follow-up appointments with my ENT, which I have every three months, are billed at $600 each. It is easy to see how the entire cost of my treatment was somewhere between $225,000 and $250,000.

I was lucky to have good insurance and am extremely thankful for that. My out of pocket cost for my treatment was around $2,000. Many people who need treatment are not so lucky. I hear stories from other survivors of how they lost their homes, had to file for bankruptcy, ruined their credit and/or will now be in debt for the rest of their lives.

If this isn't hard enough, there are additional financial considerations. What if you can't work during treatment? Some people are still able to do so, but I wasn't one of them. I honestly don't know how people can work during treatment.

I was fortunate in that I was able to take four months off to concentrate on taking care of myself. My wife was able to use family leave through her work and take ten weeks off to help take care of me.

Most hospitals and/or clinics will work out payment plans. I still don't believe this is enough. The financial aspects of this disease can be devastating. This fact is something else not discussed a great deal. And the expenses do not end with the last treatment. Follow up appointments and dealing with the long-term side effects creates long-term ongoing expenses. I will have follow-up exams for at least the next five years and medications and supplements for probably the rest of my life.

I find medicine a particularly odd industry when it comes to costs. There is no other industry in our society that I can think of where you are not told the costs of a product or service before you decide if you want it. You would not use a mechanic who took your car and said, "I don't know what the cost will be or what I am going to repair until I am done. Then I am giving you a bill that doesn't explain what I did. It will say something like 'car repair'. I will then make up a number, and that is what you will pay."

But that is how the costs of medical services work. When I did happen to ask what an appointment, test, or procedure would cost, medical personnel usually had no idea. My doctors were not aware of how much was charged for anything they did.

During my cancer process I received hundreds of EOB forms (Explanation of Benefits) from my insurance company where the date of service, type of service, and cost of service is supposed to be outlined. These rarely made sense. The providers were often people or organizations I did not recognize and the service that was provided was not clear. It might say "outpatient surgery" or "supplies" without explanation as to what these actually were. Next to the service, there was some arbitrary number that was the amount charged. Sometimes the EOBs would not arrive until months after the date of service, so I would have no recollection as to what it was for. I participated in so many appointments, saw so many professionals, and had so many procedures that it was impossible to track.

I believe that this medical billing chaos is created by the insurance companies. There are universal codes, at least in the United States, called CPT codes (Current Procedural Terminology) that are used to report medical and diagnostic procedures and services to insurance companies. For example, if someone comes in to see me for an individual therapy session and I spend 55 minutes with the person, I bill insurance using the CPT code 90837. This code tells the insurance company that the service was psychotherapy for 53 to 60 minutes.

Here is where the chaos and confusion begin. There are many different insurance companies, and it is the insurance company who decides what amount will be paid to a provider for each specific CPT code. For the code I used for illustration above, no two insurance companies will necessarily pay the same amount for the same code. One insurance company may pay $70 for that code while another may pay $200. They say they base the reimbursement amount on what they consider a "usual and customary rate," but honestly it seems arbitrary.

For the work that I do, I contract with about a dozen different insurance companies and only use two or three different CPT codes. Even with this, I cannot track who pays what amounts for what codes. Amounts also tend to change each year.

Physicians and other medical providers may work with dozens of different insurance companies and use dozens of different CPT codes. Each code has a different reimbursement rate, and the rates will vary by insurance company. One visit to a physician can include services that are billed under many different CPT codes. The codes can be very general, so instead of explaining what the outpatient services were, the insurance company may use the classification of "outpatient services" and offer no further explanation. This is what the patient sees on the EOB, a statement that says "outpatient services" with a cost, the date of service, the provider, the allowed amount, what the insurance paid, and what the patient owes.

As a patient, the reality is that I usually will not know what I have to pay until after the fact. Even then, it is almost impossible to determine how some of the costs were assessed. I would suppose that the only way to understand the latter would be to request copies of a service provider's case notes, and the original insurance billing for each EOB. As I said, I received hundreds of these EOBs and literally could spend hours trying to figure them out.

If this is not complicated enough, each insurance company has its own rules about deductibles, co-insurance, and client copays, which will vary from individual to individual even under the same plan. The rules will also vary by CPT code or type of medical provider and whether or not the provider is in network or out of network. There are so many variables that the system creates mass confusion for everyone involved.

I have called insurance companies and asked what their reimbursement rate was for a specific CPT code that I was going to use in my practice. It is not unusual that they cannot tell me. A typical answer is "we don't know until we receive the bill and review it."

It is frustrating to me when I see people trying to raise money for treatment and see the profits that pharmaceutical companies report. I wish I had some answers for those who cannot afford care. It is a huge issue, one of many having to do with cancer. Sadly, it is not a priority in our society, and for whatever reason, we have accepted a system that often causes financial hardship and makes no sense.

It is difficult to obtain accurate numbers regarding the costs of research, development, marketing, and manufacturing of cancer drugs. However, what is not disputed is that pharmaceutical companies make huge profits. These profits are in the millions and sometimes even the billions. This amount of profit is made after the costs of research and development, manufacturing, and marketing are subtracted.

An article, published on January 4, 2019, in an online medical journal called JAMA Network Open, studied the cost of research and development of ninety-nine cancer drugs approved by the FDA from 1989 to 2017. This cost of research and development for each drug was then compared to the profits gained by the companies that developed them. The study found that median income return by the end of 2017 was $14.50 for every $1.00 of research and development spending. The return range was $3.30-$55.10 of income for every $1.00 spent on research and development.

In 2018, the amount of money that pharmaceutical companies spent on marketing their drugs was estimated to be $30 billion dollars. Of this amount, $20 billion was used to persuade physicians to prescribe their drugs.

The American Cancer Society states that one of their goals is to raise money for research to ultimately find a cure for cancer. They donate around $145 million dollars per year for cancer research. This donation, which is a result of fundraising campaigns where donations often come from cancer survivors and those close to them, represents less than one percent of the marketing budget for pharmaceutical companies. Pharmaceutical companies can well afford to put more money into finding a cure for cancer.

Again, it makes no sense to me that we organize and

participate in bake sales, fundraisers, and public events to raise money for cancer research when there are billions of dollars of profit already being made by the companies that are supposed to be advancing the research.

Yet we still accept that there isn't enough money to work toward a cure. We should be putting our energies into regulating the costs of cancer drugs and creating a system where treatment is affordable. We believe the pharmaceutical companies when they claim their expenses for research and development are so high that they cannot reduce the cost of drugs to the consumer. However, they make millions of dollars in profit while presenting an image as if they are "in it" with us patients, fighting to find a cure. Cancer is an industry. Corporations and individuals become rich because of it.

PART II

CHAPTER 12
THE PSYCHOLOGICAL IMPACT
OF DEALING WITH CANCER

According to the Head and Neck Cancer Foundation, one in four cancer patients will experience clinical depression and/or anxiety as a result of their cancer diagnosis and treatment. Trauma-related reactions, which I will talk about in detail later in this chapter, are also common. I believe that the number of cancer patients who experience mental health issues is far greater than any study suggests.

Dealing with the psychological impact of my cancer and treatment was as challenging, if not more challenging, than dealing with the physical impact. Just as the physical effects of cancer and treatment can be complex and unpredictable so too can the psychological effects. Responses such as denial, fear, anxiety, depression, and anger are a few of the common psychological reactions to cancer, and each individual will have his or her own unique response. It is also possible that psychological healing can take longer than physical healing and it is harder to measure. You can see physical wounds. You can't see psychological ones.

The intensity, duration, and severity of the psychological impact of the cancer process will vary and depend on a number of factors. As mentioned previously, these factors include an individual's personality, coping style, medical diagnosis, type of cancer, duration and side effects of treatment, and support system.

Psychological issues can and often manifest long after treatment has ended. In fact, the full psychological impact of the cancer process often is not experienced until an individual is well into recovery. This was something that was never discussed with me by any professional during or after treatment.

There is not a cancer survivor I have spoken with who has not experienced or continues to experience the psychological impact of this disease. And yet this is still barely discussed, if it is discussed at all. We readily acknowledge and treat the physical aspects of cancer. We tend to ignore or invalidate the psychological ones.

It is important to have an understanding of what may happen psychologically as a result of cancer and treatment and what can be done if it becomes problematic. The key phrase here is "if it becomes problematic". Feeling angry, depressed, anxious, and fearful are normal reactions to cancer. However, when these issues begin to negatively impact relationships, work, or otherwise cause distress, they may not resolve on their own without help.

Potential mental health issues should be discussed as possible side effects of cancer and treatment along with the possible physical side effects that are discussed. The psychological impact of the cancer process should be continually assessed and treated, just as the physical impact is continually assessed and treated.

From my personal experience as a cancer patient and my experience meeting other cancer patients, the need for better psychological care is real. This need is not a new discovery. A study conducted in 2013 and published in the Cambridge University Press concluded that sixty-eight percent of head and neck cancer patients reported unmet psychological needs during their cancer process.

> *"The results of this study highlight the overwhelming presence of unmet psychological needs in head and neck cancer patients and underline the importance of implementing interventions to address these areas perceived by patients as important."*

I do not believe this is the first study to come to this conclusion, and I don't believe it will be the last. Now in 2019, six years after this study, the psychological needs of head and neck cancer patients, or of any cancer patients, in most places remains unmet.

The lack of mental health care and support throughout the cancer process is an avoidable tragedy. Throughout treatment and recovery, it was extremely rare for a medical professional to inquire as to how I was feeling emotionally. There were and continue to be many questions about my physical health. Is there any pain in my neck? How are my taste buds? Are there any lumps or changes to my throat that I have noticed? Rarely, if ever, is there a question regarding my mental state.

I have noticed this trend with friends and family as well. Well intended, and genuinely concerned, ninety-nine percent of the people who ask how I am doing are specifically asking about my physical condition. How does my neck feel? Are my taste buds back? Can I drink beer again? The only people who would even think to ask about how I was doing emotionally are either cancer survivors themselves or people who work in the mental health field and are familiar with trauma.

There are likely many reasons for the lack of assessment and treatment of mental health issues during the cancer process. To begin with, our culture does not deal well with emotional issues (just look at how many mass shootings there have been by individuals who couldn't find a better way to deal with their anger, frustration, and pain). Most people have not experienced facing their own death. We tend to avoid thinking about it, talking about it, and supporting others who are dealing with it. We don't want to acknowledge our own mortality and historically will go to almost any length to deny it—until we are faced with it.

It is also not realistic or reasonable to expect a medical specialist, such as an ear, nose and throat doctor or oncologist, to assess and/or treat mental health issues. Even if they were willing and able, there is the real issue of how busy they are. My medical oncologist stated that she is always "drowning in patients". There are far more cancer patients than there are professionals to serve them. This seems true everywhere whether it is a large or small facility or a rural or urban area. To add other duties to an already maxed out practitioner is not practical.

It may also be difficult for the medical community and cancer patients themselves to acknowledge and understand that the process of dealing with cancer and treatment can create long-term psychological consequences. We tend to think of trauma as something resulting from violence, a natural disaster, or combat. It may take some rethinking for our culture to accept that facing cancer and treatment, or possibly any life threatening or debilitating disease, can be as traumatic of an experience as any other deeply distressing event.

Still, there should at least be an information and referral process where patients can be linked to mental health professionals and/or peer support. Social workers and/or mental health counselors should be part of treatment teams. And there definitely needs to be better communication to patients regarding mental health resources and potential mental health issues. Referrals can be made to mental health professionals who work outside of the cancer centers, or the cancer centers can hire social workers and include meeting with them as part of standard medical appointments. At the very least, cancer centers and/or medical offices can provide information regarding the psychological aspects of dealing with cancer.

The cynic in me believes the lack of assessment and treatment of the psychological aspects of cancer is primarily a money issue. Specifically, the issue is profit. As previously stated, cancer is a hugely profitable industry, especially pharmaceuticals. Consumer spending on cancer drugs was estimated to be $207 billion dollars in 2015 as reported by the IMS Institute for Healthcare Informatics. During that same year, consumer spending on anti-depressants and anti-anxiety drugs, as reported by BCC Research, was around $29 billion dollars. Consumers spent $178 billion dollars more on cancer drugs than on drugs for depression and anxiety. Clearly, the drug market for cancer is much more profitable.

In an article from *The Journal of Oncology Practice* titled, "High Cancer Drug Prices in the United States: Reason and Proposed Solutions," the author pointed out that "In 2012, 12 of the 13 new drugs approved for cancer indications were priced above $100,000 per year of therapy." That is roughly $8,300 per month for a single cancer medication.

A quick online search shows prices for common anti-depressants and anti-anxiety medications range from $15 to $50 per month. There seems to be no financial motivation for the assessment and treatment of mental health issues during the cancer process.

Another sad issue regarding mental health treatment is that we tend to devalue mental health treatment in this country. If you doubt this, just look at how the movie and television industry portrays mental health therapists. Therapists are usually portrayed as having a multitude of serious mental health issues themselves and regularly crossing professional boundaries (i.e. having sex with clients or having other types or relationships with their clients outside of the office setting). I have yet to see a show or movie where a mental health therapist was the hero or even valued as a professional.

Our mental health system endures constant budget cuts, closures of institutions that care for the mentally ill, and more regulations regarding service access and the types of services that can be provided. There always seems to be a shortage of services or an inability for individuals to access services due to cost and/or availability.

In my personal experience as a mental health provider, I have seen and experienced a yearly reduction of the rates that insurance companies will pay for my services, more regulations regarding what insurance will and won't pay for, and increased regulations as to how and what mental health services can be offered. In effect, these regulations override a provider's professional judgment. There has also been an increase of paperwork required by insurance companies. Over the past year and a half, two of my primary referral sources have increased their paperwork requirements while simultaneously reducing their reimbursement rates by twenty-five percent.

In the city where I practice, most insurance companies currently reimburse me at about $95 per hour for a 55 to 60-minute therapy session. My 15 to 20-minute appointment with my ear, nose and throat physician who asks me how I am doing and looks in my throat, is billed at $620. If my ENT sees three patients in an hour, he can bill $1,800 for an hour's work. Even if the insurance company only pays half of this, he is still paid nine times more per hour than I am.

I understand that a physician has had more years of training and schooling than I did. However, to do my job I had to complete a master's degree (six years of college), 3200 hours of supervised training post-graduate school (two years), and then pass two state licensing exams. Like a physician, I also have to pay for office space, a billing specialist, licensing and continuing education fees, and general and professional liability insurance.

I can't help but wonder if mental health issues related to cancer, or for that matter any mental health issue, would become a priority if pharmaceutical companies found a way to profit as much from mental health as they profit from cancer. I would predict that mental health concerns would become a primary focus.

I do want to acknowledge there has been some progress being made in dealing with the mental health aspects of cancer. Large cancer treatment centers, such as Cancer Centers of America and MD Anderson, do indeed have staff and programs that focus on mental health. There is a field of specialty called psychiatric oncology, also referred to as psycho-oncology, which deals specifically with the psychological factors relating to cancer. Large treatment centers have psychiatric oncology units that are staffed by psychiatrists, psychologists, and social workers. However, these programs are still few and far between, and in my opinion, late in coming. Cancer centers that are smaller, which still make up the majority of cancer treatment centers in the United States, either don't have these programs at all, or they seem to be in the infancy stage of development.

My frustration is that the process of Western medicine acknowledging and addressing mental health issues as they relate to cancer is extremely slow, inefficient, and severely lacking. This is in spite of years of studies as well as years of anecdotal evidence (just talk to a cancer survivor) that clearly illustrate receiving a cancer diagnosis and/or going through treatment can be as taxing on the psyche as it is on the body.

It also seems that when we do finally begin to acknowledge the psychological needs of cancer patients, we treat it as if it is new discovery and a new process. It feels like we continue to reinvent the wheel. In my geographic area, there is some movement toward addressing psychological needs. However, when I talk to the professionals who are involved in this process, services appear as if they are being developed from scratch. Advisory and exploratory committees are being formed, and needs discussions are beginning. On the surface this all may appear to be progress. However, there already are programs in the U.S. (and I would assume in Europe) that have been designed to meet the psychological needs of cancer patients. Why doesn't the local center spend time investigating how the other larger centers are addressing the psychological needs of their patients? Again, centers like MD Anderson and Cancer Centers of America have departments that address the psychological needs of cancer patients. Why aren't we working with them to determine what works and what doesn't and look at starting similar programs if existing ones are of value? Instead, we work in a vacuum, starting over and moving slowly, and destined to make mistakes that may otherwise be avoided if we would only explore what is already out there.

The psychological issues that may occur as a result of the cancer process can be successfully treated. However, these issues first have to be identified, acknowledged, and discussed. Then they have to be addressed. Assessment and treatment of mental health issues as they relate to cancer and treatment should be as much of a priority as assessment and treatment of the physical aspects of the disease. If only.

CHAPTER 13
GRIEF

BELIEVE THAT THE majority of possible psychological issues related to the cancer experience can be classified as either grief reactions or trauma responses. In 1969 a psychiatrist named Elisabeth Kubler-Ross proposed five stages of grief. These stages were originally introduced as the way individuals deal with death and dying. However, it is possible that grief reactions can occur in a variety of other circumstances, including when it is discovered that you or someone you care about has cancer. The five stages of grief proposed by Elisabeth Kubler-Ross are:

- Shock/Denial
- Anger
- Bargaining
- Depression
- Acceptance

These stages do not necessarily occur in a clear linear fashion and limiting grief to five stages may not be all inclusive. For example, anxiety can be a big part of the grieving process as well and can manifest as agitation, desperation, fear, panic, and even anger. The stages can be viewed as more of a guideline for understanding, accepting, and working with grief issues.

More often than not, an individual bounces around

between the different stages of grief or may be experiencing more than one stage at a time. For example, when I was diagnosed, I was still grieving the loss of my mother, who died five months earlier. My father died unexpectedly three days before I was diagnosed. Then my cancer diagnosis sent me into shock, denial, fear, and anxiety. I was experiencing many stages of grief simultaneously for different reasons.

It is important to understand that experiencing the stages of grief is normal and necessary for healing. Grief doesn't feel good, and because of that fact, it is our inclination to try to shut it down. This only complicates it, potentially making it worse. Grief is a necessary process where the psyche is ultimately working to heal itself. When someone has not completely grieved a loss, more severe psychological issues can occur. I work with many people where healing means they must grieve and experience the stages of grief that were never experienced before. This is how they become unstuck.

There is no prescribed timeline for grief. Grief reactions will come and go. Even though it is a normal process, it does not mean that help is not necessary. There are therapists who specialize in grief work. There are grief support groups, and there are many books and articles on the subject.

During the cancer process, the first stage of grief, denial/shock is likely to occur as soon as cancer is suspected or when the diagnosis is given. Denial is our psyche's way of protecting itself. We hear the diagnosis and recommendations, but at the same time don't totally believe it is true. This is when we question the correctness of the cancer diagnosis. This is when nothing makes sense. This is when we say, "This can't be happening," and wish it was all a dream.

I definitely experienced both shock and denial when I was informed of my diagnosis and prognosis. I was told I had throat cancer and without treatment I would likely die an unpleasant death in four to six months. Though I clearly heard my doctor say this, there was a part of me that thought he was wrong. I felt fine, so it must have been a mistake. It was just some cruel joke that someone was playing on me. I spent the next several days walking around in an altered state, like somehow I had left my body. I kept waiting to wake up, but it didn't happen. It was real.

After the reality started to sink in, I became fearful and angry (Stage 2). Why me? What did I do to deserve this? I was angry at my ENT for discovering it. I was angry at myself and believed I somehow caused it. I was angry at my parents because I was sure they had something to do with it. I was angry at my body for betraying me. I was angry at my faith and at the world. I was also terrified. I was not ready to die. I wasn't ready to deal with treatment. I didn't want to live with the long-term negative side effects. There was no good choice. I had to choose between options I didn't want. It was not fair.

I started thinking things like, if I can make it through this easily, I will be a better person. I will do things differently. I will take better care of myself. I will find religion, give away my belongings, help the poor and needy...and so on. Maybe there is an easy cure, and if there is, I promise I will be different. I will be worthy of being saved. This was stage 3, the bargaining phase.

I dealt with feelings of depression from the time I was diagnosed and even after I was cured (stage 4). First, I thought I would die. When I learned about the treatment, I feared it would be as bad or worse than death. It would be torture, and I would not be able to escape it. I felt hopeless. I felt trapped. I believed I would never have a normal life again. Even before starting treatment, I had difficulty sleeping, and I was tired all the time. I had trouble concentrating and had little appetite, all symptoms of depression.

The acceptance phase of the grief process (stage 5) is still a work in progress for me. I find it extremely difficult to accept everything that has happened. Maybe a better way to put this is that I am having difficulty coming to terms with it all. I have made strides in this area but still struggle. Sometimes it seems like it never really happened. Then I look in the mirror and see the scars on my chest from the port and the feeding tube, and I see the area across the top of my chest and neck where hair will no longer grow due to the radiation treatments, and I am reminded that my experience was real.

Grief is complicated. It is not an orderly process, and there is not a prescribed duration of each stage. I might feel depressed for minutes, hours, days, or months and then find myself back in denial, bargaining, or feeling helpless and angry. This is not uncommon.

After my diagnosis, my world changed. My hopes and dreams, my routines and rituals, my goals and focus, what was important and not important, and my sense of self, were all turned upside down. Nothing felt solid anymore, and nothing would ever be the same.

Throughout the cancer process, I grieved many losses. My body changed. I lost thirty-five pounds, lost my muscle tone, lost the hair on my face, neck, and chest, lost my ability to eat, lost my energy, and lost my ability to think clearly and stay alert. My face thinned. My senses were altered, and I didn't recognize myself in the mirror. My focus in life became one pointed—to survive. This meant taking medications, managing my feeding tube, going to treatment, attending medical appointments, and having lab tests. My new life was totally different than anything I had ever experienced before.

I could not eat or drink and could barely swallow. I had a six-inch tube that protruded from a hole in my stomach. I carried a backpack with a feeding pump in it. I had a metal disc, or port, implanted under the skin of my chest. I was heavily medicated most of the time, couldn't drive, and did not feel good. My new identity was that of cancer patient. Every record about me, every appointment, and every test was identified by my birth date first. I was now patient 5/9/1963. I had lost myself and was grieving this loss. I had no idea if the me I knew before would ever return.

Along with depression came anxiety. I worried all the time. I worried about if I would have side effects or pain or if treatment would work, if I was ingesting enough calories, if I would be cured, or if I would soon die. I worried about being a good patient, being a bad patient, and what my future would be like if I even had one. I worried that I was a burden to my wife, who was taking care of me, and wondered how helpless she must have felt.

I lived not in the present, but for my future, believing that once I was finished with treatment I would feel better emotionally. This was not the case. It wasn't until after I stopped treatment, had my feeding tube removed, and received the news that my cancer was gone, that the full impact of what I had been through really hit me.

All at once I started experiencing the grief of my father's death, the grief of my friend Fred's death, and the trauma of my cancer. I don't think there was room for me to do this until recovery. Before completing treatment, I was so focused on surviving each day and my daily routines and on managing side effects, that I shut down a large part of the emotional impact. Denial is a survival mechanism, and I was trying to survive.

CHAPTER 14
TRAUMA

A TRAUMA IS THE experience of a deeply distressing or disturbing event. Being diagnosed with cancer and going through treatment can certainly be traumatic. A traumatic event or events can have a major impact on our ability to function in the world.

Never, from the beginning of the diagnosis phase to where I am now over a year post diagnosis, have any of the dozens of medical professionals whom I have seen used the word trauma. Yet every head and neck cancer patient I have spoken to readily acknowledges some level of trauma that their cancer and their experience with treatment and recovery has caused. Every aspect of the cancer process—receiving a diagnosis, preparing for treatment, participating in treatment, recovering, and dealing with short- and long-term side effects—can be a traumatic experience.

I experienced the entire cancer process as traumatic. During the phases of diagnosis, preparation, treatment, and even recovery, I experienced and continue to experience some level of psychological distress. Since my initial diagnosis of cancer, I would say I have dealt with grief reactions, clinical depression, anxiety, and trauma responses. This is not uncommon, and sadly, it is also not uncommon for these issues to go unaddressed.

How a trauma experience manifests and when it manifests is somewhat of a mystery. For example, I have worked with combat veterans who initially experienced few symptoms of trauma. Then, without explanation, years after a traumatic event, something is triggered. These veterans begin experiencing severe symptoms of trauma that negatively impact their daily lives and relationships.

The way our psyche operates sometimes creates a delayed reaction to stress. During cancer treatment, there is so much to focus on during the cancer process that sometimes the psyche cannot handle it all, so in effect it shuts down anything psychologically painful. It is like the psyche puts anything too difficult to deal with into a box, which then is carried around. This box may stay closed, may leak at some point, or may burst open.

All trauma responses tend to share some similarities. In my case it was somewhere around five months into my recovery that I started experiencing nightmares, anxiety, constant thoughts about death, and was triggered by anything related to cancer. These are common issues after experiencing a traumatic event.

Imagine drawing a long horizontal box on a piece of paper. Now imagine that inside the far-left side of the box there are very few, if any, trauma symptoms. Inside the far-right side of the box, there are many severe symptoms of trauma. So, as you move from the left side to the right side of the box, the number and severity of trauma symptoms increases. As the number and severity of symptoms increases, the psychological distress and the negative impact on social and/or occupational relationships also increases. Someone experiencing the symptoms of trauma may fit anywhere on this continuum, and the severity and intensity of symptoms may also change.

POST-TRAUMATIC STRESS DISORDER

Post-Traumatic Stress Disorder (PTSD) is probably the most widely recognized trauma diagnosis. This diagnosis is given to an individual who experiences a severe response to a trauma (or traumas), which manifests as a collection of symptoms that causes psychological distress. The length of time that symptoms have occurred, and the number and severity of the symptoms, will determine if someone is diagnosed with PTSD. This does not mean that individuals who have experienced a trauma will always develop PTSD, but people who do develop PTSD have always had one or more traumatic events that have caused it.

According to a study published in January of 2018 by the American Cancer Society, about one in five cancer patients will develop PTSD (diagnosed about six months after the initial cancer diagnosis). The study went on to conclude that one-third of these individuals who were diagnosed had persistent or worsening PTSD four years later. Again, I believe the numbers are higher than what is reported.

The American Psychiatric Association states:

"People with PTSD have intense, disturbing thoughts and feelings related to their experience that last long after the traumatic event has ended. They may relive the event through flashbacks or nightmares; they may feel sadness, fear or anger; and they may feel detached or estranged from other people. People with PTSD may avoid situations or people that remind them of the traumatic event, and they may have strong negative reactions to something as ordinary as a loud noise or an accidental touch."

Types of experiences that can cause PTSD include a vehicle accident, a natural disaster, extreme violence, or anything where you feared for your life or someone else's. The experience of cancer and treatment can also be the cause of PTSD. Someone who supports a cancer patient (a friend, spouse, family member, or medical professional) can also develop PTSD, or lesser trauma symptoms, by witnessing and/or being part of the process.

The mental health profession currently groups trauma symptoms into four categories:

- Arousal
- Negative Mood
- Avoidance
- Intrusions

Below are common symptoms that may be experienced in each category:

Arousal Symptoms: difficulty concentrating, sleep issues, a heightened sense of being on guard, living in fight or flight mode, and experiencing a long-term heightened state of general anxiety.

Negative Mood: agitation, anger, numbness, extreme emotional expression or little or no emotional expression, guilt, blame, inability to remember significant events or parts of events, and lack of interest in activities. A person may be "stuck" in strong emotions (horror, shame, sadness) or appear and/or feel disconnected.

Avoidance Issues: avoidance of talking about the trauma or anything related to it, making light or minimizing the trauma or the symptoms caused by the trauma, avoiding places, people, things, or TV shows that bring back memories of the trauma, and avoiding feelings and thoughts that relate to the trauma.

Intrusions: frequent thoughts of death, nightmares,

re-experiencing and/or replaying the trauma, and psychological and/or physical reactivity to reminders of the traumatic event, such as an anniversary of the event.

People who experience PTSD may engage in self-destructive behaviors, become violent, have poor impulse control, and develop other issues, such as generalized anxiety and/or depression. They may not trust anyone, isolate themselves, end or "blow up" relationships, become suicidal, and/or engage in high risk behaviors. An eating disorder can develop as well as other physical problems. Alcohol and drug use and abuse are common for individuals who have PTSD.

Individuals who have experienced trauma often react to triggers. A trigger is a stimulus that evokes feelings, thoughts, or memories of a trauma. A trigger may be a sight, a smell, a sound, a place, a thing, a person, or an activity. The reaction to a trigger can include anxiety, anger, confusion, fear, and panic. Sometimes individuals are aware of their triggers, and other times they are a complete surprise. It can feel like living on a roller coaster.

I treated a veteran who had recently returned from a tour of duty in the Middle East. He used to have panic attacks when he saw a cardboard box on the road. While he was in the Middle East, he had been part of a convoy, and when they drove past a cardboard box, it exploded. He was injured, and some others were killed. Memories of his trauma are triggered when he sees cardboard boxes, and he becomes extremely fearful and anxious.

Treatment for issues related to trauma typically includes learning coping skills and recognizing and learning to deal with triggers. Treatment also includes allowing an individual to process the emotions associated with the trauma, in a sense allowing the grieving process to occur. Sometimes medication is needed to help stabilize the individual while new coping skills are learned and emotions are processed.

MY TRAUMA REACTION

Up until treatment ended, I was so busy every day that I could only focus on what was directly in front of me. When treatment ended, I no longer had one full day each week dedicated to chemotherapy sessions. I no longer had daily radiation and hydration appointments, and my doctor and lab visits were fewer. I was told I needed time to heal but was given little to no guidance on how to do this other than to rest. I would not know for at least three months if the treatment was successful because testing sooner than this could produce invalid results.

Physically, I felt my worst when my treatment ended. After six weeks of radiation and chemotherapy, all of the cumulative side effects hit me. I was the most tired, the most nauseous, my throat was the rawest, and the skin on my neck was burned and peeling. I became severely anemic, and my white blood cell count was too low. Within a week of finishing my last radiation treatment, I was in the emergency room because I was running a fever. I was admitted to the hospital. I felt abandoned by my team, who had left me with little instruction as to how to heal physically and no instruction on how to heal emotionally.

After I was discharged from the hospital, I started seeing a naturopath. Unlike my other doctors, my naturopath had several ideas on how I could help my body heal after treatment ended. She was the person who realized that a big part of my not feeling well was a long-standing intolerance to the feeding formula I was ingesting. She helped me with recipes for homemade feeding formula, encouraged me to stop using my feeding tube when I slept to give my body a rest, and started me on several herbal supplements. I am convinced that without her assistance, physical recovery would have taken much longer and been much harder.

I am not sure what I expected from recovery. I had not thought a great deal about it. I had assumed that soon after treatment ended, I would feel a sense of relief and somehow things would go back to the way they were before treatment. Not true.

After treatment, my last hospitalization, and my port and feeding tube removal, I wasn't sure how to process everything that had happened. Physically, I was finally feeling better and experiencing increased energy. The pain in my throat subsided. My taste buds were returning. I had only minor physical side effects from my treatment. This included an altered sense of taste, dry mouth, some swelling in my neck, and some minor difficulty swallowing due to scar tissue in my throat, the result of the radiation.

Though I was healing physically, I seemed to feel worse emotionally. For a number of months, I felt confused, anxious, and depressed, and started exhibiting more symptoms of a trauma response. I was having nightmares and anxiety attacks, and instead of feeling hopeful for my future, I was scared and pessimistic.

I felt very alone. Most people who knew me figured I was now better given that "I was cured" of cancer, and since I looked and felt better physically, most people thought it was all over. The outpouring of support diminished as people assumed I was now fine and went on with their lives. I never assigned any malice to this. This was understandable. Emotional scars cannot be seen, and unless someone has been through a trauma or worked closely with people who have, it is extremely difficult to understand the impact. This is further confused by the fact that often the full impact of a traumatic event takes time to surface. Here I was, five months post treatment, cancer free, and feeling emotionally distraught.

I should have been feeling happy and thankful that I was alive and healthy again. Instead of joy and gratitude, I was full of fear and guilt. How do I explain to others that I feel guilty about surviving cancer? How do I justify my existence when there are so many good people who won't survive cancer and so many bad people who will never get it? Why did I survive while others did not and would not? None of this made any sense to me.

I was hard on myself. I told myself my experience was not that bad, and I shouldn't have any issues as a result. Why was I even writing about it? Who was I to presume that my story was even worth telling? I had cancer. I got treatment. I got better. What is the big deal? I was just spoiled and needed to get over myself.

I had this standard in my head about how I should feel post cancer. Like in the movies, the world was supposed to be brighter, food was supposed to taste better, the birds would sing more, every day would be sun and roses, and...it wasn't so. In many ways I was more confused, more frustrated, and more disillusioned. The cancer process was like someone took me out of my world, turned it inside out, shook it around a bit, reorganized and reshaped it, and then put me back in it without a map.

I still got angry when stuck in traffic. I still got annoyed and impatient with others. I still complained. These were things I was never supposed to do again because I had a second chance, a new lease on life. I was supposed to come out of my cancer process as a new and enlightened person, having unlimited compassion for others and an appreciation for life that others would see and admire. This is how I wanted to be, hoped to be, and strived to be.

But there have been only brief glimpses. There are moments where I experience what true appreciation and presence feel like—a genuine connection to the universe. Then, I try to grasp at it to make it last, and it slips away—and I am reminded that I am only human.

Given some time and distance from my cancer and treatment, as well as professional and peer support, my emotional state is slowly improving. The nightmares have become rarer, and I don't feel as hopeless. I can think a little into the future now whereas before I had trouble thinking past the next day.

The hard part about trauma is that there is no way to predict how long it may or may not impact someone. It can be triggered at any time, often unpredictably. There can be good days and bad days or even good moments and bad moments. However, dealing with trauma can become more manageable and less intense and not necessarily interfere with living life. I'll take that as a win.

FEAR OF RECURRENCE

Recurrence of cancer is a real possibility and depends on a number of factors, including the type of cancer and the type of treatment. After treatment ends, it is normal to fear that cancer may return. Milestones, such as the anniversary of starting or ending treatment, periodic checkups and testing, or a host of other things, can trigger this fear. It is when the fear and worry negatively impact our lives that help may be necessary.

Ultimately, we cannot control whether cancer returns or if a new cancer develops. We can only control how we react to the information. I don't believe that indulging a fear of recurrence is helpful. I also realize this is easier said than done. I have been extremely fearful at times during my recovery. The week prior to each one of my throat checks, I have difficulty sleeping. I worry and constantly think about what I would do if my cancer returned. I know this fear and worry are not helpful, but that does not mean it is easy to eliminate. It only serves to rob me of the present moment. It is not possible to enjoy what is happening now if I am worrying about what might happen tomorrow.

When we are talking about the fear of cancer recurrence, we are not talking about having to process emotions that have been blocked. There is no benefit in indulging this fear or allowing yourself to fully experience it. In fact, some of the information you will find about dealing with fear of recurrence encourages distracting yourself from it. This is the opposite of what needs to happen to process trauma. For trauma to resolve, we must move into the emotions. In dealing with fear and worry regarding the recurrence of cancer, it can be helpful to distract yourself and thus avoid the emotions.

What can also be helpful is being aware of your fear, talking about it, and looking deeper to see what might be behind it. Behind the fear of recurrence often lies other issues: fear of death, fear of leaving this earth with regrets, fear of pain or discomfort, or fear of leaving family behind. These issues could be helpful to explore. By coming to terms with whatever drives our fear of recurrence, we can decrease the worry and fear associated with the possibility of cancer returning. This will likely take time and may require the assistance of a mental health professional.

A TRAUMA INFORMED APPROACH

Over the past several years, the U.S. Department of Health and Human Services has been developing what is now known as a "Trauma Informed Approach" or "Trauma Informed Care".

According to the Substance Abuse and Mental Health Services Administration (SAMHSA, which is part of the U.S. Dept. of Health and Human Services):

> *"When a human service program takes the step to become trauma-informed, every part of its organization, management, and service delivery system is assessed and potentially modified to include a basic understanding of how trauma affects the life of an individual seeking services. Trauma-informed organizations, programs, and services are based on an understanding of the vulnerabilities or triggers of trauma survivors that traditional service delivery approaches may exacerbate, so that these services and programs can be more supportive and avoid traumatization."*

I have several years of professional experience working with people who have experienced traumas, including veterans with PTSD, and I have to admit I had never heard the term, trauma informed care, until a few years ago. I don't believe any of the medical professionals whom I saw during my cancer, treatment, and recovery were familiar with trauma informed care. Yet the goal of SAMHSA is to educate and train all human service organizations on this approach. Obviously, something needs to be done differently because the information is not reaching those who need it.

To be honest, when I first read about a trauma informed approach, I didn't think much of it. It wasn't that I didn't believe it was important, it just seemed somewhat obvious to me. Though I had never heard of trauma informed care, I believed I was sensitive to issues relating to trauma and had a pretty good grasp of how people responded to trauma in their lives. It was not until I experienced being a cancer patient and doing more of my own research on what a trauma informed approach might look like, that I developed a deeper appreciation and understanding of the concept. After I had a greater understanding, I realized there is a huge need in our medical system for this perspective as well as training for medical personnel on what this actually means when providing services.

One of the experiences I shared earlier in this book was when I had become so frustrated and overwhelmed that I stopped using my feeding tube and was not eating or drinking. When I saw the radiation oncologist and he noticed I had lost around fifteen pounds in a week, he said in a loud critical tone, "How about a little cooperation here?" He didn't even make eye contact with me, rather he was looking at my file.

His way of handling this situation was the opposite of a trauma informed response. A trauma informed response to my situation would have been his consideration of the possibility that I was experiencing my cancer and treatment as a traumatic event. I was only a few weeks into treatment and having difficulty adjusting to my new life. I was frustrated, scared, angry, and anxious. I felt ill and weak. I was having difficulty with my feeding tube and feeding formula and felt as if no one was helping me with this issue. I reacted to all of this by shutting down and avoiding (common responses to trauma), which for me translated to not eating or drinking and pretty much pretending that things were normal.

I was not doing what I was supposed to do, and I was making decisions that were causing myself harm. The non-trauma informed approach to a situation like this is to ask the question, "What is wrong with you?" That is exactly what I heard when the radiation oncologist insisted I cooperate. What was wrong with me that I could lose fifteen pounds in a week? In his view I needed to be reminded of the consequences of not complying with what he believed was best for me, and somehow this was supposed to motivate me to change my behavior.

When approaching someone as a trauma informed provider, the question is not "What is wrong with you?" but rather "What happened to you?" What would have been the outcome of our meeting if the radiation oncologist would have put down my file, looked at me directly, softened his eyes, and said something like, "Jeff, it looks like you lost fifteen pounds this week. What do you think happened?"

I then could have told him what was really going on. I could have told him I was lost, scared, confused, and angry. We could have worked together to find a solution. I would have felt validated, empowered, and listened to. I would have likely complied with his recommendations to use my feeding tube and pump after realizing I was not thinking clearly. Most importantly, I would not have felt like my interaction with him was yet another of a string of traumatic events that kept occurring.

It would not have taken any more time for him to respond to my situation differently. It also would have likely led to a better outcome for both of us. As it was, this particular radiation oncologist was only filling in for a short time, and I never saw him again.

The only reason I started using my feeding tube and pump again was due to the nurse navigator, who was also at this meeting. She intervened and calmed the situation down. She shared her concerns with me in a gentle, caring, non-judgmental manner. She probably had not realized it, but her way of handling the situation with me was exactly what a trauma informed approach would involve. She seemed to understand that my behavior and my choices were not motivated by my desire to be oppositional or non-compliant but resulted from my experiencing a real traumatic event in my life, and therefore I was not thinking clearly. I was only a few weeks into treatment, but the trauma of my cancer process, physically and psychologically, already had a real impact on my feelings, thoughts, and behaviors. A trauma informed approach seeks to understand, not to condemn.

POST TRAUMATIC GROWTH

As I previously stated, issues related to trauma can be treated and the symptoms effectively managed or eliminated. Given time, some individuals experience something called post traumatic growth, also referred to PTG.

Individuals who experience post traumatic growth often report that as a result of dealing with a traumatic event, they have gleaned benefits. These benefits typically include a greater appreciation of life, closer family and friend relationships, and a reorganization of life's priorities. Often, individuals report feeling a new strength and an ability to facilitate and cope with change better than before.

It is hard to think about gleaning benefits from cancer. Yet I have experienced some of the aspects of post traumatic growth. Overall, I do have a greater appreciation of life. Many of my relationships have become closer, and my priorities have changed. I know there have been times when I was fearful of something and I thought, "I made it through cancer treatment, what I am worried about now is really no big deal."

There are also times when I experience the more difficult aspects of trauma. I can hope that these more difficult aspects will dissipate, and the post traumatic growth aspects will expand. It is interesting to simultaneously be thankful and appreciative and bitter and angry about the same experience.

CHAPTER 15
SUGGESTIONS FOR CARING FOR YOUR EMOTIONAL HEALTH

H ERE ARE SOME suggestions based on what I learned from my cancer process about my own emotional health. I hope it can be helpful to others.

1. Do not fear your emotions.

This can be difficult for some people. There is no correct emotional response. There is no correct way to express whatever emotions you might feel, and there is no timeline for doing so. Your emotional reaction may be huge and "off the charts," or it may be muted and seemingly nonexistent. Your feelings may change over time or sometimes change in an instant. Feeling angry, frustrated, anxious, happy, and sad are all normal. Though all emotions are normal, this is not necessarily a license to be mean to others, especially the people who are trying to help you. Remaining kind to others during the cancer process can be challenging.

2. Don't compare yourself with how you used to be.

The cancer process will change you. Just as there may be long-term physical issues, there may be long-term psychological issues as well. You may experience a new normal physically, and you may experience a new normal psychologically. I am still trying to figure out my new normal, both physically and psychologically. Comparing my reactions to things, my mental stamina or toughness, or even my view of the world, to how I was before cancer is not helpful. It also doesn't make sense most of the time. I have to remind myself of this. Sometimes I find myself thinking, "I used to be able to deal with that better," or "That used to not bother me." I have to remember that my reality is not the same anymore. Things trigger me that never used to. I feel things at a deeper level. I become confused and mentally fatigued easier than I used to. These may or may not be permanent issues, but for now they are part of what is real for me. Lamenting over what I used to be able to handle or deal with just makes it harder.

3. Don't compare yourself to others.

Undoubtedly, you will meet others in various stages of the cancer process. Some may be just beginning while others may be longtime survivors. Just as everyone's physical health will differ, everyone's mental health will differ as well. I know cancer patients who may have a bleak treatment prognosis but have a more positive attitude than I had or do. I start to wonder what is wrong with me. Then I beat myself up even more than the cancer did. Again, not helpful. My mental state is my own. My issues are my own. Comparing my mental state with others does nothing positive for me. It only creates self-criticism and guilt.

4. Find support for your emotional health as well as your physical health.

I hope by now I have made the point that dealing with your emotions is important during all phases of the cancer process.

Support is paramount, and the more the better. Friends, relatives, peer groups, and professionals are all resources that I used, and I needed them all. There is no correct timing for seeking out support. Maybe there will be emotional impact right away that needs to be dealt with, and maybe it will happen a year after treatment ends. Like everything else in this process, there is no right or wrong.

5. Focus on your own emotional needs first.

During your cancer process, you would not choose to inflict additional damage to yourself physically, so why risk doing damage to yourself psychologically? What I am suggesting is not having unsupportive, toxic, and/or negative people around you. I don't see any upside to keeping those types of relationships. You may lose friendships or relationships, but my experience is that I have formed new relationships or intensified relationships that already existed. Not everyone will know how to deal with your cancer. Some people will be insensitive and unsupportive and even tell you horror stories about others in similar situations. When someone is not helpful, it is not worth having that person around. It does not have to be permanent. You can always reconnect later if you want to, but if your focus is on truly healing, why add to the toxins that will already be put into your body?

6. Ask for help and support and accept it.

This is harder for some than for others. I have found that most people want to help but often don't know how. Sometimes I had to give someone clear instructions— "I don't want any advice or problem solving. I just want you to listen to what I have to say."

Finding a professional or more than one to talk to was invaluable. Once I discovered that it was available to me, I met weekly with an oncology social worker, had regular meetings with the nurse navigator, started attending a support group for head and neck cancer survivors, and found a good therapist. Again, you will have a medical team, why not have a psychological team as well?

7. Educate yourself.

Talking to others who have been through what you are experiencing can be extremely helpful (assuming you are dealing with positive, supportive people). Learn about the psychological issues involved in dealing with the cancer process. Understanding depression, anxiety, grief, and trauma can help you identify what might happen and plan strategies for coping. Many times throughout this process, just understanding that my emotional experiences were normal was helpful in and of itself.

8. Remember, nothing is permanent.

At times during my experience, it felt as if nothing would ever change. Whatever happens to you, it will pass and change. That is the nature of things. Everything is impermanent. I found this often hard to remember, but it was comforting when I was reminded. No matter how bad I felt, it would pass.

9. Find something positive that will occupy your mind.

During the cancer process, it is easy to go to dark, negative places in your mind. It is not helpful to feed fear, worry or regret. Finding something else for your mind to do can be helpful. For example, fantasizing about food was a great way for me to distract myself from going to some dark places. Sometimes it is as simple as bringing your focus to your breathing, and every time your mind wants to venture into darkness, bring your focus back to your breath.

I recall one instance during treatment when I felt very discouraged and depressed. My wife started asking me the meaning of some Spanish words. We had both been working on learning Spanish since we enjoy going to Mexico. At first, I was resistant to answering her questions but soon played along. I realized later she pulled me out my darkness by giving me something else to focus on. It was something I really appreciated and at the time didn't even realize it had helped so much.

I believe that as part of recovery, it is important to find things that help you stay present. For me, I have found some hobbies/activities that help me to focus on what I am doing in that moment. When I am focused on what I am doing in the moment, I forget about cancer and death, and I even forget to worry. Training the mind to be present can be as much work as training the body for a sport. It is a process that takes time, energy, and effort.

10. Build yourself back up physically.

When you feel better physically, you feel better mentally. Cancer treatment changes you physically and taxes all of your systems. Before treatment I was running and working out regularly. I was not able to exercise during treatment. I didn't have the energy (of course, if you can exercise during treatment, it could only help). I remember walking to the mailbox and being tired. However, as soon as I was able to after treatment, I started back to the gym with the help of a personal trainer. I remember only being able to sit in a chair and lift up each leg ten times before I was exhausted. But I kept coming back and slowly working on things. Eventually, I was able to run again and do whatever type of exercise I wanted.

In addition to exercise, I have been taking supplements recommended by my naturopath and eating a healthy diet. I have been working on building my insides back up as well. I believe that feeling better physically helped my mental state tremendously.

11. Rest.

The cancer process is physically and emotionally exhausting. Resting the mind is as important as resting the body. A few months after my treatment ended, I decided I should be ready to resume some normal activities, pushing myself through my fatigue. This wasn't a good idea. I needed more rest than I was giving myself. For several months I needed ten to eleven hours of sleep per night. This did change eventually, but I had to honor what my body and mind were telling me.

I notice some changes in my mental focus. I have trouble focusing if I see too many clients in a day whereas this wasn't such an issue prior to treatment— part of my new normal.

Some survivors will deal with physical and/or emotional stamina issues long-term. Fighting whatever reality you experience regarding your physical and emotional stamina only causes healing to slow and doesn't change anything.

12. Stop fighting your new normal.

It is our nature to seek pleasure and avoid pain. Just as there might be short- and long-term physical side effects of cancer, there will likely be short- and long-term psychological side effects as well. Fighting them, being angry about them, and refusing to accept or acknowledge them only makes them worse. I have noticed I still occasionally have nightmares and can become anxious or sad when talking about cancer or attending my cancer support group. I still become angry when I talk about some of the aspects of treatment and recovery that I really hated or thought should have been handled differently. I still worry. These things may change over time, or they may not. I am doing what I can to help myself process my experience, but the reality may be these are things I have to live with and learn to manage.

Physically, for example, one consequence of my treatment is that I have had some hearing loss and now wear hearing aids. I don't relish this idea. I have struggled about some of my beliefs around this. I believed hearing aids were for older people and I might be judged as being disabled or less capable because I have to use hearing aids now. I don't like the fact that treatment impacted my hearing. I am angry at the fact that no one had discussed with me hearing loss as a potential side effect of treatment, and no one suggested I have my hearing tested once treatment ended. I also realize that none of this would have made much difference. My reality is that my hearing was getting worse. If I want to hear better, I have to wear hearing aids. I could spend energy railing against this idea, but that does not change my reality. The choice that causes me the least amount of suffering is to accept it. Just as I must accept that my psychological responses to situations may be different now as well— and acceptance does not mean I have to like it.

To summarize, the cancer process is likely to include some psychological distress. Throughout the cancer process, all thoughts and feelings are normal, and there is no single way to deal with them. Though normal, these thoughts and feelings may still cause distress, and help may be needed to deal with the issues that arise. It is also likely the medical community will barely address the psychological impact or not address it at all. If you are in distress, seek help. Take care of yourself and be gentle with yourself. You can learn new coping skills and process through your emotions. Strive for acceptance of the reality of your situation, which doesn't mean you have to like it.

CHAPTER 16
RECOMMENDATIONS FOR SYSTEM CHANGE

THE FOLLOWING IS what I believe needs to be included as part of the cancer process for the psychological impact of cancer and treatment to be adequately addressed:

- The assessment and treatment of psychological issues are included as part of all stages of the cancer process.

- Medical professionals should be trained in trauma informed care and recognize when patients are experiencing symptoms of mental health issues. Appropriate information and referral services should be available to patients and their families.

- Social workers and/or other mental health specialists should be an integral part of treatment teams. Referrals to this type of professional should occur during the initial diagnosis process.

- Mental health follow-up services (e.g. check-ins, assessment, and/or treatment) should occur at least as long as physical follow-up services continue. Mental health resources and services should be available indefinitely for cancer patients and their families/loved ones.

- Survivorship plans (plans for how to live healthfully after treatment) should be developed for all patients and include goals and objectives for the management and improvement of psychological issues.

- Written and verbal information should be provided regarding the psychological impact of cancer and treatment, including information regarding the grief process, trauma, anxiety, depression, and fear of recurrence. This information needs to be available to the patient as well as the patient's care provider(s)/family members.

- Care providers and loved ones of the cancer patient should be educated about the potential psychological impact that they may experience. They should also be made aware of the mental health support they might utilize.

Depending on where you receive services, some or all of these things may be occurring. My experience included almost none of the above. Rather than waiting for the medical community to better address the psychological needs of cancer patients, I believe that we as patients need to be the catalyst for change. Fair or not, it is ultimately up to us to advocate for ourselves and each other. The first step, which I have tried to illustrate, is understanding the potential psychological impact of the cancer process. Understanding this will help us recognize our needs, and when we know what our needs are, we can start conversations with our treatment team about how they might be met. We are our best advocates.

I would hope that at some time in the near future cancer treatment centers would adopt policies, processes, and procedures that would include all of things I have mentioned. I don't know of any spokesperson for any cancer center who would deny that a holistic approach to cancer treatment is beneficial. It is past time to implement this belief. Dealing with the psychological aspects of cancer is not a new idea. There are resources and models of how to do this that likely could be copied. It does not have to be complicated or costly, but it does have to be important.

CHAPTER 17
COMPASSION

C OMPASSION IS A true caring about someone else's circumstance, the ability to understand someone else's pain, and the desire to help. It is the opposite of blame, judgment, control, cruelty, apathy, or indifference.

Compassion was something else that was not discussed during my cancer process. I have come to believe the practice of compassion for oneself and others is extremely important for healing and recovery. At every step of the process, there were opportunities to practice compassion for others and for myself.

I expected a certain amount of compassion from others. That only made sense. I had cancer. However, the real challenge was for me to have compassion for myself and others who I encountered during my cancer process. This included having compassion for other patients, friends, family, and medical professionals. This was especially difficult when someone was not so compassionate toward me.

It is not uncommon for a cancer diagnosis or any life altering circumstance to trigger an egocentric response. My focus and my world shrank. I became the center of my own universe. Call it ego, call it biology, or call it survival, it all has the same outcome. Everything was about me, and I became extremely self-focused. After my diagnosis, it seemed as if every waking moment was about my life, my cancer, my treatment, my pain, and my world. My needs and priorities trumped everyone else's.

Sometimes it felt like I was "holding an ace in the hole." At any time, I could play the cancer card and expect that all attention would shift to me. But… but… but… I have cancer. It usually worked. I got all the attention.

Shortly after treatment I attended a showing of a documentary about terminal illness. At the end of the movie, we divided into small groups of five people and discussed our thoughts about the movie. The documentary was impactful and difficult. When it was my turn to talk, I shared I was only a few months post cancer treatment. I remember feeling the weight of this admission, and the seriousness, and maybe even feeling sorry for myself. I expected sympathy and got it.

It was then that I noticed an older couple in the group. The man was well-dressed and had an air of sophistication and pride. There was a small oxygen tank on wheels sitting on the floor next to him. I had not noticed this earlier since I was absorbed in my own process.

During the time when we talked about the movie, he didn't say much. After the group task was completed, I made an effort to talk to him. I liked his energy and he seemed kind. He and his wife had moved to this area to be closer to their grand-children. They were living at a local assisted living facility, and he continued to work in his own consulting business about half-time. He had COPD (Chronic Obstructive Pulmonary Disease), late stage, with a bleak prognosis. The COPD would eventually take his life. It was only a question of how much time he had left.

I felt stupid, ashamed, and humbled. This man was dying and didn't say much about it. I was cured and still feeling sorry for myself. I had been so egocentric that I could not see anything or anyone but me. I had lost my perspective and my compassion.

There is a delicate balance here. On the one hand, to survive, I had to be self-focused for a period of time. There were so many things I had to do to get ready for treatment, survive treatment, and recover. This required an egocentric response. But the more egocentric I became, the less compassionate toward myself and others I also became. I do not believe this is a healthy state of mind nor one that is conducive to healing.

So why is being compassionate important? To answer this, let me start with addressing compassion for oneself. I had talked about my crisis of faith and how I wondered if somehow I had created my own cancer. Was it karma? Something I had done in this or a previous life that was the cause? For a time, I felt as if I must have done something terribly wrong and deserved cancer. Even though I couldn't identify what it was, I still must have done something. This self-judgment was the opposite of having compassion for myself. It was like being shot with an arrow and then inserting another one at the same point of entry. Self-judgment only increased my suffering.

I noticed a lack of compassion for myself was an ongoing problem. Even after treatment when my cancer was gone, I feared I didn't deserve to be cancer free. There was no way to win. By not being compassionate with myself and by being self-critical and judgmental, I was keeping myself from moving forward and truly healing.

For me, the art of self-compassion is to allow myself to feel what I feel and think what I think without self-judgment and without allowing these thoughts and feelings to control me. Putting it another way, it is not fighting my emotions or thoughts, but not letting them dictate my behavior either, just recognizing and acknowledging them, and then letting them rest.

This is easier said than done, and lacking compassion for my own situation only made it worse. Beating myself up did not make anything easier and did not and does not work as a motivator for healing. Whether I deserved cancer or didn't deserve it, or deserved to heal or not to heal, was irrelevant. I felt how I felt, and I could choose to fight it, to do battle with myself, or to accept it.

We often are our own worst critics. We say things to ourselves that we would never say to anyone else. I would never tell someone just to "get over it" after experiencing a traumatic event. Yet that is what I have told myself. All this did was make healing from whatever emotional wounds that remained, more difficult.

Self-compassion is about being gentle with myself. That means accepting those parts of myself that I may not necessarily like. It means accepting that I was and still am lucky to now be cancer free while acknowledging that others are not so lucky. It means accepting that I don't have answers to the many questions that I still have and that I don't understand the randomness of this disease. The sooner I can learn to be gentle with myself, to approach my own pain with compassion instead of condemnation, the sooner I will heal.

Throughout my cancer process, I was reminded that I needed to practice compassion toward others as well. This included having compassion for medical professionals, caretakers, friends, family, and even strangers.

The majority of medical professionals whom I worked with were amazing. Given the number of appointments I attended weekly, I must have dealt with more than a dozen professionals each week. There was the radiation oncologist's office and staff, the medical oncologist's office and staff, the infusion center staff, the physical therapist, the speech therapist, the social worker, the nurse navigator, the X-ray technicians, the hospital and emergency room staff, my primary physician's office, surgeons, wound care staff, the ENT and his staff and assistant, and various other physicians and medical staff I encountered. Most of these professionals saw ill people all day, every day. I can't imagine what it must be like to spend all day, every day, with cancer patients.

At times it was easy for me to forget how hard of a job these people have. On top of dealing with many patients, they are often short staffed, and they work with patients who are in bad moods, who sometimes act out their frustrations on them. They have insurmountable paperwork to complete and often must make decisions that could mean life or death for someone. The stress of those jobs must be incredible.

There were times when the professionals whom I dealt with were not so cheery or downright rude. I felt angry more than once at some of these individuals who seemed to not care. There is something satisfying about righteous indignation— "How dare you be rude to me, I have cancer. Don't you get it?"

I also remember a number of professionals who made the extra effort to connect with me. Sometimes it was just for a few seconds to ask me how I was doing or to tell me it would all be okay. There were dozens of people who were involved in my treatment and recovery process, so many more than I would have thought, and I remember almost all of them. I remember those who were kind and assuring, and I remember those who were detached and cold.

As I thought about what their days must look like, I started seeing the professionals as more human. They have their struggles just as I was having mine. In fact, I remember one infusion nurse telling me she was going through breast cancer treatment while she was working. I remember feeling confused. She was one of the professionals. She wasn't supposed to have any issues herself; she was supposed to be there to help me.

Yet there she was, going through cancer treatment and having to continue to work at the same time, and she did it with a smile on her face. I will say it again, if for no other reason as to remind myself, we ALL have our struggles and challenges.

When I completed my treatment, I made sure that I sincerely thanked the people who were involved who literally had saved my life—my ENT, medical oncologist, radiation oncology staff, the nurse navigator, the social worker, and the staff at the infusion center that supplied my feeding tube supplies. This was not everyone who participated, but these were the primary people for me. I wanted them to know how much I appreciated their kindness even though many of them didn't remember me. I was one of many whom they served every day.

When I would forget how hard their jobs were, I could become agitated about not getting the attention I wanted or having to wait a few minutes for someone to come help me with something. I could be less than compassionate with the people who were there to help me and who had extremely difficult jobs. It was okay for me to feel frustrated and impatient at times, sometimes with good reason, but it was not okay for me to be rude or disrespectful to those who were helping me. This can be a hard practice to remember.

Being compassionate toward my wife, who was my primary caretaker, was important to me. I have witnessed cancer patients being mean and disrespectful to their caretakers, usually their spouses, out of frustration and feelings of helplessness. This is one of the reasons I suggest professional help (e.g. a therapist) as strongly as I do. Feelings of frustration, anger, and resentment are all normal and expected. However, for me, this does not excuse or justify treating someone poorly. It doesn't make sense for me to yell at, be rude to, or belittle the person who is taking care of me. In some situations, it is the person I might not survive without. It is okay to feel whatever you feel. You can be angry or upset or have negative feelings. However, I do not believe that it is okay to act these feelings out in a negative way and potentially hurt the people who love us and the people who are helping us. Processing these emotions with a professional can save relationships.

Of course, being kind to others applies to friends as well. The reaction that friends and acquaintances had to me and my cancer surprised me at times. Some people, whom I would not have expected to, really stepped up and helped. Some people wanted to help, but either didn't know how to or didn't know how to be supportive. These people will simply assure you that everything will be okay or say things like "Well, you just have to go through treatment," and often these people believed that once treatment was completed, everything was over and there was no reason to talk about cancer anymore.

These people were often the great "task" people. The fact that they wanted to help, but seemed to do it somewhat awkwardly, made them perfect (at least they were in my case) for assigning specific tasks to do. The tasks included anything from providing transportation to picking up groceries. I didn't expect these people would provide me with emotional support, but they were there for the tasks that needed to be done and their intentions were pure.

There were even people who decided on a task on their own and then completed it. I had an acquaintance, who I had only met a few times, insist on cleaning our roof gutters. This was his way of showing that he cared. I thought this was great.

There were also people who were friends or acquaintances who disappeared after they found out I had cancer, or given their reactions, they were people I chose not to include in my life anymore. I believe this is normal as well and attribute this mostly to what happens when we are confronted with our own mortality. Some people cut and run when the topics of death and disease are openly discussed.

There were times when I felt hurt and disappointed by the people who either disappeared or at least seemed to distance themselves from me. I initially took it personally. Then I realized it ultimately was not about me, that something in them couldn't deal. I shifted from frustration to compassion. This does not mean I would want some of these people back in my life, just that I could let go of my resentment.

The key here for me is that lack of compassion for others ultimately holds myself hostage. If I am angry, frustrated, acting out, and reacting to everything, I make myself miserable. Holding onto anger typically hurts me more than anyone else. Acting out of anger can permanently damage relationships.

So, how do you embrace compassion for yourself and others throughout the cancer process? I found that realizing that everyone has challenges in their lives, and everyone has a story, was extremely helpful. This was most obvious when meeting others in treatment. I could become so self-focused during my process that I would forget about the struggles of others. Yet all I had to do was attend one of my chemotherapy appointments to see many others who struggled as well.

The first time this really hit home for me was when I started a conversation with a young man whom I had seen receiving chemotherapy each time I was there. He was always alone, and I never saw anyone come to see him. His treatments took the entire day as did mine. He had testicular cancer, and he was twenty-five years old. He seemed understandably despondent.

I had no idea what his story was; we engaged in small talk. But I realized I felt bad for him. I felt bad that he didn't have anyone with him when he was receiving his treatment. I felt bad that he had to deal with cancer at such a young age, and I felt bad that there was nothing I could do except to acknowledge him and be kind.

I saw people have adverse reactions to chemotherapy drugs that were being administered. I had conversations with people who were terminally ill with cancer and receiving chemotherapy in an effort to extend their lives a little longer. I talked to people who had neuropathy (a common side effect of chemotherapy) so bad that they had difficulty walking, and there were those who would likely be receiving chemotherapy treatments for the rest of their lives.

Then there was me—the lucky one. My chemo treatments were only once a week for six weeks. My wife was always there with me. I had friends visit and sit with me. I experienced no immediate side effects during my chemotherapy drug injections. I never experienced neuropathy.

Having compassion for others can be difficult. Feeling someone else's pain is never pleasant and experiencing true compassion for others going through the cancer process was and is painful. However, for me, there is something sacred about being part of someone else's journey. It is a connection with another human being that is beyond words. I believe true compassion is something that transcends this realm of reality. It is a reminder that we are more alike than we are different. It helps me heal and gain perspective. It releases me from my own egocentrism, and it ultimately reminds me that perhaps the meaning of life can be very simple, that we are here to help each other.

Compassion for myself is similar. Allowing myself to feel my own pain without judgment, without fixing, and without apologies, was and still is difficult. Yet I believe true compassion for oneself is also sacred. I am convinced compassion comes from my higher self. This is the me that is not self-centered, judgmental, or critical, but rather the me that is gentle and kind to myself and others. It is the me that meets the world with an open heart.

I don't believe that we can be compassionate to anyone else until we can be compassionate with ourselves. Without exception, I have discovered that during the times I am most critical and judgmental of others are the same times I am the most critical and judgmental of myself. In contrast, those times I am most compassionate with myself are the times I am most compassionate with others.

A friend of mine and I were talking about his wife who was dealing with treatment and complications related to breast cancer. He made a comment about seeing the beauty in suffering. I did not understand this. If someone would have said to me that there was beauty in my suffering when I was in the middle of my treatment, I might have lashed out at them.

As I thought about this, it made a little more sense to me. The first thing I realized is that without pain, we would not understand pleasure. Without suffering, we would never understand joy. If we only know one side of things, one perspective, or one experience, and there is no opposite experience for comparison, how can we grasp or appreciate the meaning? It is the yin and the yang. We would not understand darkness without light. If it was always dark, we would not know any differently, and we would never understand or appreciate the light. Without suffering we cannot see, understand, or appreciate joy.

I have come to understand just how much suffering opens our hearts. The people I have met in my life whom I have truly admired are those who had suffered greatly at some time in their lives. They were able to transform their suffering into joy, compassion, and presence. We see this in the stories of Christ and Buddha. We see this in great role models, such as Martin Luther King, Gandhi, and Mother Theresa. The commonality is that each of these individuals suffered greatly, and each of these individuals transformed this suffering into amazing compassion.

I have a long way to go to be this type of person. My journey has given me the desire. It is a start.

CHAPTER 18
GRATITUDE
AND GIVING BACK

I T IS DIFFICULT to think about being grateful for cancer. I wish I had never had it. I wish I had never been through treatment. Yet here I am. And there are many things I am grateful for. First and foremost, I am still alive. I made new friends, and I have a new perspective on life. At present my health is probably better than it has ever been. The long-term side effects of my treatment are minimal, and I can easily live with them.

I realize I have an important choice here. I can be bitter and resentful about my experience—about having to live with a diminished sense of taste, hearing loss, a non-functional thyroid, and some loss of physical and emotional stamina— or I can appreciate what I have learned from my experience and that I am now healthy and alive. This is indeed a choice. Sometimes it doesn't feel that way. Sometimes I still go to dark places.

I had little control over my experience of cancer and treatment. I could not predict or direct how the treatment would impact me physically or emotionally, but I always had control over what I did with this information. Ultimately, my attitude and my behavior were and still are my choice.

I am not saying it is healthy to stuff and deny feelings.

There will be anger, resentment, and fear. In my opinion, these emotions must be honored and acknowledged in order to heal, but I don't have to live in these emotions. They don't have to be the constant driving force of my life. Once I have explored, experienced, and given them the attention they demand, I can let them go. Of course, this can be a difficult process that takes practice and time, and for me it is still a work in progress.

I am so grateful to the people who helped me through this process. I experienced love and support in ways I have never experienced. Without dealing with cancer, I may never have experienced that in quite the same way.

I discovered that I have a strong desire to give something back to this world. I wish I could say my motivation was purely altruistic, but that would not be true. To be honest, there are many motivating factors, and some even possibly involve feeling guilt about recovering from this disease while others do not. Regardless, I find I want to help others. Exactly what this looks like, I don't yet know. It may be as simple as doing my best to be nice to people daily. I know that writing this book was one of those ways I wanted to give back. As I stated in the introduction, if there is even one thing that someone going through cancer (or a support person helping someone going through it) can glean from this that eases suffering, even a little bit, then I believe I have accomplished something. I wish I would have had better guidance throughout my process, especially regarding the psychological aspects of this disease and what to do when treatment ended and recovery began.

One last thing I wanted to mention regarding giving back; it does not have to be cancer related. One of the ways that actually makes the most sense for me as a way to give back would be to see cancer patients in my therapy practice. I have thought about this, and maybe one day I will. However, right now I am not ready. I am still too close to my experience to remain objective and not be triggered. Even in writing this book, some sections were hard to relive. In the end, however, I am convinced it helped with my healing.

There are many ways to give back to this world, and I am confident I will find ways that work for me. I believe this is part of my obligation to others since I survived. Helping each other in this world has no downside.

I have no doubt that my experience has become part of my identity. I am many things: a man, a therapist, a son, a husband, a brother, a writer, and a cancer survivor. My cancer experience is part of my identity, but it is does not define who I am. My journey continues. I wish you the best on your journey. You are not alone.

EPILOGUE

IT HAS NOW been two years since my official diagnosis, and I am still cancer free. In the course of writing this book, some of the issues regarding how local services are delivered to cancer patients, and some of the issues regarding feeding tubes, have improved.

I had discussed the fact the radiation oncology center in this area was owned and operated by a non-profit organization and the medical oncology center was owned and operated by a for profit company. This is changing. The non-profit organization has purchased the infusion center and is planning to expand and build a three-story cancer center where all needed services will be located under one roof. This means that all laboratory, imaging, pharmaceutical, nutrition, and other support services, will be located in one place. This was not the case when I went through treatment. Every appointment I had typically meant traveling to a different location.

The new cancer center will also employ additional social workers and nurse navigators, provide private spaces for infusion patients if desired (instead of having treatments in a large room with several other patients nearby), and provide meeting space for doctors or other professionals who might come to the center to see patients. There will be rooms provided for support groups and the availability of massage therapy.

When I no longer was using my feeding tube, I had several boxes of unused feeding formula that I wanted to donate, but I had difficulty finding a place that would take them and make them available to another patient. The new center will provide storage for donations and distribute donated items to patients who need them. This will be a huge help to patients.

The start date for the construction of the new cancer center is early 2020. In the meantime, a social worker and a nurse navigator have been added to the team at medical oncology, whereas before they had none. There is now better coordination of services, particularly around issues related to feeding tubes. They have stopped inserting the type of tube that I used. Recall that I had to be put to sleep, and the tube was run down my throat, into my esophagus, through my stomach, and then out my abdomen. The tubes they use now are called jejunostomy (J) tubes. They are inserted into stomach through the abdomen while the patient is under conscious sedation. This procedure is much easier and safer. A 'J' tube is easily removable by deflating a balloon behind the abdomen wall. Once the balloon is deflated, the tube slides out. The opening of the tube can remain flush with the outside of the abdomen. Recall that mine stuck out about six inches and frequently would catch on things.

Within forty-eight hours of a 'J' tube being inserted, a patient attends a workshop on how to use and care for the feeding tube. Patients are also immediately referred to the wound care clinic so that they may begin a relationship with the staff there in case there are any issues with the feeding tube or the stoma, the area where the tube exits the abdomen.

This is all a great start in making needed systemic changes. Though there are still other issues that need to be addressed, these changes represent major progress in our local service delivery system for cancer patients.

The nurse navigator, who was new at her job when I started treatment, followed me throughout my process. In a recent conversation with her, she jokingly told me that she saw many "opportunities for positive change" while she observed my experience. I had many conversations with her about issues I was having or had during treatment, and she has been an excellent advocate for changing processes and procedures that would better benefit cancer patients. I am forever grateful that she continues to help cancer patients. Anything that can help make this experience a little easier is a huge step.

Personally, things continue to change for me as well. My hypothyroidism is finally under control with the correct dosage of medication. Finding the correct dosage took some time and some experimentation. I have become accustomed to my hearing aids. The current hearing aid technology is amazing, and I can use them to hear and talk on the phone and stream music and podcasts through them.

A pleasant surprise for me has been the continued improvement in my sense of taste and saliva production. Only a few weeks ago was the first time that a bowl of fruit tasted good to me. This was almost twenty months after treatment ended. More foods are tasting better, and I appreciate the taste of food so much more.

Psychologically, I feel better as well. Though I still struggle at times, I feel less angry about my whole experience. I can allow myself to think about the future. I am much more aware of my own mortality and still think about death frequently, but I have less intrusive thoughts and nightmares are infrequent. Occasionally I am still triggered by some things, usually cancer related. I do believe that when I am triggered, the impact is not as severe and does not last as long. This is all good news.

Though I would love to avoid talking about, thinking about, or being around cancer, I find that this is not the case.

My journey has given me some insight and understanding that I believe I need to use to help others. Instead or running away from all things cancer related (which is what my mind says I want to do), I find myself moving toward them, and even providing support to others who are dealing with cancer and treatment. This is hard. I lost another friend to cancer last year. I have other friends who are struggling with various stages of cancer. Before I was diagnosed, dealing with cancer was never a part of my life. I rarely ever thought about or talked about cancer. Now it is a daily part of my life. I find myself dealing with my own issues which resulted from cancer and treatment, being with or talking to friends who have cancer, or talking about cancer with others.

My new normal is still hard to identify, constantly changing and unfolding. I understand better than ever that things are not solid and static. What is today may not be tomorrow or the next day. I realize that it is my job to accept this fact—that what is normal is that there is no normal.

APPENDIX 1

Below is a summary of what was involved in my cancer process:

OVERVIEW

Thirty-three radiation treatments to my neck while masked and bolted to a table

Six chemotherapy treatments (eight hours each, one time per week for six weeks)

Two hospitalizations (one for dehydration and one for low white cell count)

One visit to urgent care for skin issues around my feeding tube

Five months using a feeding tube (unable to eat/painful to swallow/food tasted terrible)

Over 1000 cartons of feeding formula consumed

About two months of daily hydrations (two hours per day every day)

SURGERIES/ PROCEDURES

Throat biopsy

Needle biopsy of my neck

Feeding tube placement (October 2017)

Feeding tube removal (April 2018)

Port placement in my chest (October 2017)

Port removal (March 2018)

Throat scopes (Aug 2017, April 2018, July 2018, October 2018, January 2019, March 2019, July 2019, more to come)

The making of the locking mask for my radiation treatment

Dental exams/cleaning/cavity fills

Numerous blood draws

X RAYS

Head and neck

CT scan

Thyroid

Two PET Scans

Mouth X-rays

PHYSICIANS / MEDICAL PERSONNEL I SAW

Medical oncologist

Chemotherapy nurses

Radiation oncologist

Radiation technicians

Multiple radiologists

Emergency room and hospital physicians and nurses

Primary physician

Ear nose and throat doctor

Various surgeons

Nurse navigator

Dieticians

Speech therapist

Hydration nurses

Infusion nurses

Social worker radiation oncology

Lymphedema physical therapist

Lymphedema massage therapist

Naturopath

Dentist

SUPPLIES / MEDICATIONS

About eight miscellaneous medications for pain, anxiety, and nausea (liquid and pill forms)

Feeding pump with IV stand

Gauze for feeding tube hole in abdomen—changed several times per day

Stoma powder

Feeding tube belt

Tubes/bags for pump—changed daily

Bolus 60ml syringes for manual feeding

Seven to eight cartons of feeding formula per day

Fluoride trays/daily use

Spirometer (for breathing exercises)

Chew toy (for exercising jaw muscles)

Neck compression garment

SHORT TERM SIDE EFFECTS (FEW DAYS TO SEVERAL WEEKS)

Nausea

Hallucinations

Neuropathy in legs/feet (only lasted a few days)

Sensitivity to cold/chills

Sensitivity to touch

Confusion

Time distortions

Sense of smell and taste severely altered

Tired/lacked energy

Pain in throat and difficulty swallowing

Skin issues on neck

Oral thrush (lasted over six months)

Anemia

Low white cell blood count

Dehydration

Loss of sexual desire

Sensitivity to touch

Depression

Pain around stoma

Anxiety

Nightmares

Loss of weight and loss of muscle

Constipation (likely due to hydrocodone)

LONG TERM SIDE EFFECTS SO FAR

Lymphedema (swelling of neck due to lymph nodes not working due to radiation)

Taste bud changes

Limited saliva production

Sensitivity to cold

Minor throat pain due to scar tissue from radiation treatment

Trauma responses caused by the experience (improving)

Hypothyroidism (managed by medication)

Hearing impairment due to nerve damage in ears likely caused by the chemotherapy drug (now wear hearing aids)

High levels of Platinum in my system, a heavy metal resulting from the chemo drug Cisplatin (long term effects of this unknown).

OUTCOME OF TREATMENT

Excellent. I am twenty months post treatment with no evidence of cancer. My final PET scan indicated that there is no cancer in my body. The exams by my ENT show no evidence of the tumors that were in my throat. My health is very good overall.

APPENDIX 2

Post treatment recommendations: (not meant to include everything)

- Thyroid check two to three months after treatment ends, then regularly after that
- Complete blood panel after treatment ends, then regularly (every three to six months)
- Hearing exam three to six months after treatment or as recommended, then yearly testing.
- Heavy metal testing and working with professional to detox from chemotherapy drugs
- Work with naturopath regarding supplements to help immune system
- Sleep and rest (learning to listen to your body)
- Dental check soon after treatment and at regular intervals as recommended by dentist
- Primary cancer site checks, frequency determined by physician
- Detox and destress your life
- Diet and exercise (could include nutrition counseling and working with a personal trainer)
- Psychological support (could include information, therapy, or support group)

Made in the USA
Middletown, DE
19 June 2020